Self-Assessment Color Review

Feline Infectious Diseases

Katrin Hartmann

Dr med vet, Dr habil, Diplomate ECVIM-CA (Internal Medicine)
College of Veterinary Medicine
LMU University of Munich, Germany

Julie K. Levy

DVM, PhD, Diplomate ACVIM (Small Animal Internal Medicine)
Director, Maddie's Shelter Medicine Program
College of Veterinary Medicine
University of Florida, USA

D0420629

MANSON PUBLISHING/THE VETERINARY PRESS

600073608

Copyright © 2011 Manson Publishing Ltd
ISBN: 978-1-84076-099-6

A CIP catalogue record for this book is available from the British Library.

For full details of all Manson Publishing Ltd titles please write to:
Manson Publishing Ltd, 73 Corringham Road, London NW11 7DL, UK.

Tel: +44(0)20 8905 5150
Fax: +44(0)20 8201 9233
Website: www.mansonpublishing.com

Commissioning editor: Jill Northcott
Project manager: Paul Bennett
Copy editor: Ruth Maxwell/Clare Chilcott
Design and layout: Cathy Martin
Color reproduction: Tenon & Polert Colour Scanning Ltd, Hong Kong
Printed by: New Era Printing Company Ltd, Hong Kong

Contents

Preface

As a species, the cat is host to some of the oldest infectious diseases known to veterinary medicine as well as being involved at the forefront of emerging and newly discovered infections. Cats are victim to rapidly spreading pathogens and those that hide quietly within their own DNA. They have been implicated in zoonoses and the spread of infections to and from wildlife. As cats become increasingly important human companions around the world, the veterinarians enchanted by this species have developed reliable diagnostic approaches and exceptionally effective prevention and treatment strategies for many infections. Despite this, infectious diseases remain an important part of daily feline practice, either because the solutions do not yet exist or because some cats still remain outside the reach of veterinary care.

With this book, we provide an overview of feline infectious diseases in a case-based manner, the way clinicians encounter them in daily practice. We hope this practice-oriented approach motivates the reader to contemplate the cases and to reflect on how they might have managed each case.

The book was created for veterinary practitioners and veterinary students during their clinical rotations, to improve and practice their knowledge of infectious diseases. At the end of every case, questions for self-assessment by the reader are provided to test existing knowledge. The illustrations that accompany each case will help the reader to identify both classical and unique disease presentations.

We are very grateful for the expertise and hard work of all our co-authors. We would also like to thank Jill Northcott and the team at Manson Publishing for their patience and encouragement. Most of all we would like to thank our partners, friends, and colleagues in our teaching institutions for all their support and encouragement to turn this book into reality. We invite the readers to approach this book the way we approach each of our feline patients, as a series of mysteries awaiting our careful detective work in search of a happy outcome for our patients and the families that care for them. We hope that this book will inspire veterinarians to embrace the topic of feline infectious diseases and to contribute to the health and welfare of cats everywhere.

Katrin Hartmann & Julie Levy

Editor and contributor profiles

Editors

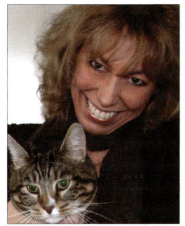

Katrin Hartmann
Dr med vet, Dr habil, Diplomate ECVIM-CA
(Internal Medicine)
College of Veterinary Medicine,
LMU University of Munich, Germany

Dr Hartmann graduated from the College of Veterinary Medicine at the LMU University of Munich in 1987, completed her doctoral thesis in 1990 and her habilitation thesis on the antiviral treatment of FIV infection in 1995. She stayed on as a Resident in small animal internal medicine, Clinical Instructor, and Assistant Professor at the Clinic of Small Animal Medicine at the University of Munich until 2001. From 2001 to 2003, she worked as an Associate Professor in the College of Veterinary Medicine, University of Georgia, USA. Since 2003, she has been Professor and Head of the Clinic of Small Animal Medicine at the LMU University of Munich, Germany. Her research is concentrated on infectious diseases in cats and dogs, with a special focus on virus infections in cats.

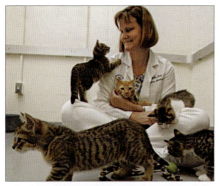

Julie Levy
DVM, PhD, Diplomate ACVIM (Small
Animal Internal Medicine)
Director, Maddie's Shelter Medicine
Program
College of Veterinary Medicine
University of Florida, USA

Dr Levy graduated from the School of Veterinary Medicine at the University of California, Davis, USA, in 1989. She completed an internship at Angell Memorial Animal Hospital in 1990 followed by a residency in small animal internal medicine in 1993 and a PhD in 1997 at North Carolina State University. Her dissertation research focused on the immunopathogenesis of FIV infection. She is Director of Maddie's Shelter Medicine Program at the University of Florida. Dr Levy's research and clinical interests center on feline infectious diseases, neonatal kitten health, humane alternatives for cat population control, and immunocontraceptive vaccines for cats. She is the founder of Operation Catnip, with two university-based feral cat spay/neuter programs that have sterilized more than 45,000 cats since 1994.

Contributors

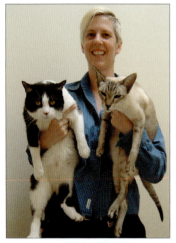

Vanessa Barrs
BVSc (Hons), MVetClinStud FACVSc (Feline Medicine)
Valentine Charlton Cat Centre, Faculty of Veterinary Sciences, University of Sydney, Australia

Dr Barrs graduated from the University of Sydney in 1990 and returned in 1993 to complete a residency in infectious diseases and small animal medicine. She attained a Master's degree in infectious diseases in 1997 and achieved Fellowship of the Australian College of Veterinary Scientists in Feline Medicine in 2000. Dr Barrs is currently Co-director of the busy feline referral service at the Valentine Charlton Cat Centre and is Associate Professor and Head of the Small Animal Medicine Unit at the University of Sydney, Australia. She enjoys undergraduate and postgraduate teaching. Her research interests include feline infectious and genetic diseases and alimentary lymphoma.

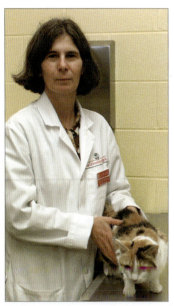

Jeanne Barsanti
DVM, PhD, Diplomate ACVIM (Small Animal Internal Medicine)
College of Veterinary Medicine, University of Georgia, USA

Dr Barsanti graduated from the New York State College of Veterinary Medicine at Cornell University in 1974. She completed an internship at Auburn University in 1975 followed by a Master's degree in 1976. She completed her internal medicine residency at the University of Georgia in 1977 and joined the faculty. Her dissertation research focused on the interaction between canine heartworm disease and the kidney. Dr Barsanti is currently Josiah Meigs Distinguished Teaching Professor, Emerita in the Department of Small Animal Medicine and Surgery at the University of Georgia, USA. Her interests focus on urinary tract diseases of dogs and cats and prostatic diseases in dogs.

Stefano Bo
DVM
Ambulatorio Veterinario Associato Bo Ferro
Nardi, Torino, Italy

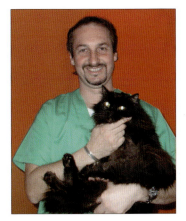

Dr Bo graduated from the College of Veterinary Medicine of Turin, Italy. From 1992 to 1994 he received a fellowship from the National Health Institute on the 'Evaluation of cats with FAIDS and its therapy'. In 1999, he completed his doctoral thesis in veterinary internal medicine. Currently he is a Lecturer at the College of Veterinary Medicine of Turin, Italy, sees patients in his private practice, and is President of the Italian Society of Feline Medicine.

Ursula Dietrich
Dr med vet, MRCVS, Diplomate ACVO,
Diplomate ECVO
College of Veterinary Medicine,
University of Georgia, USA

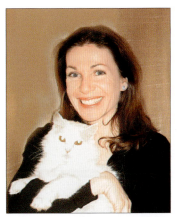

Dr Dietrich graduated from the College of Veterinary Medicine at the LMU University of Munich, followed by a doctoral thesis in ocular ultrasound at the University of Munich in 1996. She then completed a residency in veterinary ophthalmology at the University of Zurich, Switzerland in 2000. Dr Dietrich was a faculty member in the Department of Small Animal Medicine and Surgery at the University of Georgia, Athens, USA from 2001–2009. Her research interests focussed on feline and equine ophthalmology, glaucoma, and ocular ultrasound. Dr Dietrch is currently affiliated with the New York City Veterinary Specialists and lives in New York City.

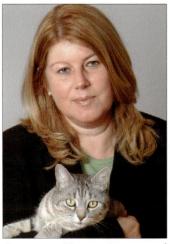

Andrea Fischer
Dr med vet, Dr habil, Diplomate ECVN,
Diplomate ACVIM (Neurology)
College of Veterinary Medicine,
LMU University of Munich, Germany

Dr Fischer graduated from the College of Veterinary Medicine at the LMU University of Munich in 1987. She completed her doctoral thesis in 1990 and a residency in neurology at University of Georgia, Athens, USA, in 1994. She completed her habilitation thesis on electro-diagnostic techniques in small animal neurology in 2000. Dr Fischer is currently Chief of the Neurology Service at the Clinic of Small Animal Medicine of the LMU University of Munich, Germany. Her main research interests focus on epilepsy, electrodiagnostic techniques, neuromuscular diseases, and hearing disorders.

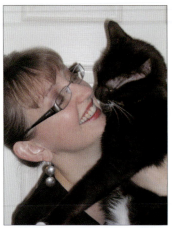

Bente Flatland
DVM, MS, Diplomate ACVIM (Small Animal Internal Medicine), Diplomate ACVP (Clinical Pathology
College of Veterinary Medicine,
University of Tennessee, USA

Dr Flatland graduated from the College of Veterinary Medicine at the University of Georgia in 1993. She then completed an internship at Colorado State University in 1994 and a small animal medicine residency and Master's degree at the College of Veterinary Medicine at Virginia-Maryland Regional University in 1997. Dr Flatland is currently an Associate Professor of Clinical Pathology at the University of Tennessee, College of Veterinary Medicine, USA, after working as an internist in both private practice and academia. Her interests include quality management, point-of-care testing, method validation/ comparison, diagnostic cytology, and pedagogy.

Patrick Hensel
Dr med vet, Diplomate ACVD
College of Veterinary Medicine,
University of Georgia, USA

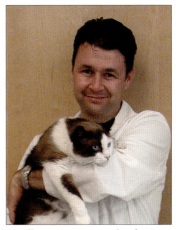

Dr Hensel graduated from the School of Veterinary Medicine at the University of Bern, Switzerland, in 1996. He completed a doctoral thesis in 2000 and an internship at the School of Veterinary Medicine at the University of Zurich, Switzerland, in 2001. He then did a residency in dermatology with board certification in 2004 at the University of Georgia, where he is currently a faculty member in the Department of Small Animal Medicine and Surgery in Athens, USA. His main areas of interest are canine atopic dermatitis, allergy testing, and infectious diseases.

Kate Hurley
DVM, MPVM
School of Veterinary Medicine,
University of California, USA

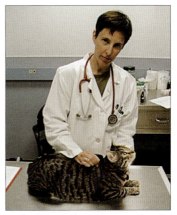

Dr Hurley began her career as an animal control officer in 1989. After graduation from the School of Veterinary Medicine at the University of California in 1999, Dr Hurley worked as a shelter veterinarian in California and Wisconsin. In 2001, she returned to Davis to complete a residency in Shelter Medicine. Dr Hurley is currently the director of the Koret Shelter Medicine Program in Davis, USA. She loves shelter work because it has the potential to improve the lives of so many animals. Her interests include population health and infectious disease, with a particular emphasis on feline upper respiratory tract infections.

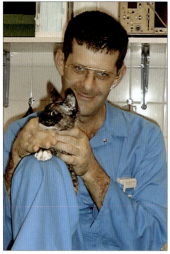

Richard Malik
DVSc, PhD, MVetClinStud, FACVSc (Feline Medicine), FASM
Centre for Veterinary Education,
University of Sydney, Australia

Dr Malik graduated from the University of Sydney in 1981. He completed a PhD in neuro-pharmacology at the Australia National University, then returned to the University of Sydney for a residency in internal medicine. He remained there for 16 years in a variety of positions, including the Valentine Charlton Senior Lecturer position in Feline Medicine (1995 to 2002). Dr Malik is currently an Adjunct Professor in Veterinary Infectious Diseases at the University of Sydney, Australia, and a Senior Consultant and Veterinary Specialist in the Post Graduate Foundation in Veterinary Science. His primary interests focus on infectious and genetic diseases, diseases of cats in general, and most recently diseases of koalas.

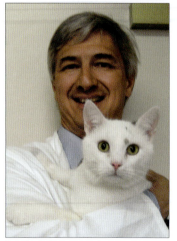

Ralf Mueller
Dr med vet, Dr habil, Diplomate ACVD, Diplomate ECVD, FACVSc (Dermatology)
College of Veterinary Medicine,
LMU University of Munich, Germany

Dr Mueller graduated from the College of Veterinary Medicine at the LMU University of Munich in 1985, and worked in private practice before completing a residency in dermatology at the School of Veterinary Medicine at the University of California, Davis, USA, in 1992. He worked in a private dermatology referral practice in Melbourne before joining the faculty at the College of Veterinary Medicine at Colorado State University in 1999. He completed his habilitation thesis at the University of Zurich, Switzerland, in 2003. He is currently Chief of the Dermatology Service at the Clinic of Small Animal Medicine of the LMU University of Munich, Germany.

Catherine Mullin
VMD, MS
School of Veterinary Medicine,
University of California, USA

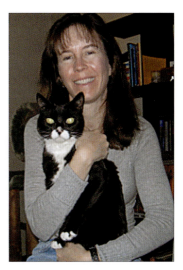

Dr Mullin received her MS at the University of Manitoba, Canada in 1988 and her VMD from the University of Pennsylvania in 1995. After an internship at the Animal Medical Center in New York City, Dr Mullin worked for the Humane Society of New York in both their shelter and low-cost clinic. Dr Mullin is currently completing a residency program in shelter medicine at the University of California, Davis, USA. She is passionate about cats, and her interests include all aspects of animal sheltering with an emphasis on feline infectious diseases.

Margie Scherk
DVM, Diplomate ABVP (Feline)
CatsINK, Vancouver, Canada

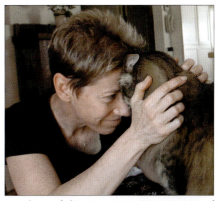

Dr Scherk graduated from the Ontario Veterinary College in Guelph, Canada, in 1982. In 1995 she became board-certified in Feline Practice by the American Board of Veterinary Practitioners (ABVP). She practiced at Cat's Only Veterinary Clinic in Vancouver, Canada from 1986 to 2008. She is the North American editor for the *Journal of Feline Medicine and Surgery* and was the President of the American Association of Feline Practitioners (AAFP) for 2007. Her interests include analgesia, ethology, and geriatric internal medicine.

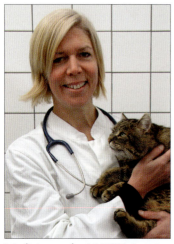

Bianka Schulz
Dr med vet, Diplomate ECVIM-CA (Internal Medicine)
College of Veterinary Medicine,
LMU University of Munich, Germany

Dr Schulz graduated from the College of Veterinary Medicine at the LMU University of Munich in 1997. She completed her doctoral thesis on feline respiratory tract infections followed by a residency at the University of Munich and at the College of Veterinary Medicine, University of Georgia, Athens, Georgia, USA, from 2001 to 2003. Dr Schulz is currently a faculty member at the Small Animal Internal Medicine Service of the Clinic of Small Animal Medicine at the LMU University of Munich, Germany. Her primary research interests focus on feline and canine respiratory tract disease, especially infectious diseases and feline asthma.

Classification of cases

Note: references are to case numbers.

ORGAN SYSTEMS

Respiratory 4, 9–11, 17–19, 25, 26, 39, 40, 42–44, 48, 52–54, 59, 79–81, 86–88, 92, 108, 109, 121, 122, 132–134, 136–138, 142–144, 149, 152, 174, 183, 184, 194–196

Dermatological 5, 13–15, 22–24, 30, 31, 35, 36, 46, 47, 49, 59, 70, 71, 75, 82, 83, 90, 91, 97, 102, 108, 109, 115, 124, 125, 129–131, 153–155, 160–163, 180, 181, 197–199

Cardiovascular 60–62, 110, 111, 116, 177, 180, 181

Urological 16, 20, 66, 100, 101, 106, 126, 127, 129, 130, 157–159

Neurological 1, 6, 7, 32–34, 38, 42–44, 76, 77, 85, 98, 99, 120, 123, 128, 135, 145, 156, 160, 161, 166, 167, 187, 190

Orthopaedic 107, 109

Ophthalmological 28, 29, 37, 69, 72, 78, 104, 105, 114, 162–164, 197–199

Oral/gastrointestinal 2, 3, 21, 41, 56–58, 63, 64, 67, 68, 84, 103, 117–119, 165, 178, 179, 186, 188, 189, 191, 193

Systemic 8, 9, 12–15, 17, 27, 45, 50, 51, 55, 73, 74, 86–89, 94–96, 112, 113, 139–141, 146–148, 150, 151, 168–173, 175–177, 182, 185, 191, 192

INFECTIONS

VIRUSES

FIV 25, 26, 46, 47, 63, 64, 67, 68, 157, 158, 166, 167, 171, 183, 185, 186, 191

FeLV 16, 33, 34, 69, 150, 151, 159, 168–170

FCoV12 32, 50, 51, 73, 74, 76–78, 94–96, 135, 148, 172, 173

FPV 2, 3, 38, 56–58, 84, 117–119

FHV 37, 184

FCV 17, 93, 184

Influenza 86–88

Rabies 190

BACTERIA

Respiratory *Mycoplasma* spp. 18, 19, 132

Haemotrophic *Mycoplasma* spp. 8

Bartonella spp. 147

Bordetella bronchiceptica 52–54, 136, 137

Mycobacteria spp. 30, 31, 46, 47, 49, 97, 140, 141, 154, 155, 174

Leptospira spp. 45

Botulism 120

Borrelia burgdorferi 107

Tetanus 1, 85, 128, 145, 187

Helicobacter spp. 21, 41, 165

Nocardia spp./*Actinomyces* spp. 22, 23, 79, 80, 92, 138

Abbreviations

ACE	angiotensin-converting enzyme	GMS	Gomori methenamine silver
AIHA	autoimmune hemolytic anemia	HARD	heartworm-associated respiratory disease
ALP	alkaline phosphatase	H&E	hematoxylin and eosin
ALT	alanine aminotransaminase	HIV	human immunodeficiency virus
ANA	antinuclear antibody	IBD	inflammatory bowel disease
AST	aspartate transaminase	ID	intradermal
AZT	3'-azido-2',3'-dideoxythymidine (zidovudine)	IFA	immunofluorescent antibody
		IM	intramuscular
		IN	intranasal
BAL	bronchoalveolar lavage	IOP	intraocular pressure
BCG	Bacille Calmette-Guérin	ITP	immune-mediated thrombocytopenia
BCS	body condition score		
bpm	beats/breaths per minute	IV	intravenous
CD	cluster determination	LDH	lactate dehydrogenase
CK	creatine kinase	LPS	lipopolysaccharide
CNS	central nervous system	MCV	mean cell volume
CPV	canine parvovirus	MLV	modified live virus
CSD	cat-scratch disease	MRI	magnetic resonance imaging
CSF	cerebrospinal fluid	PAS	periodic acid–Schiff
CT	computed tomography	PCR	polymerase chain reaction
DIC	disseminated intravascular coagulation	PLR	pupil light reflex
		PO	oral
DNA	deoxyribonucleic acid	PT	prothrombin time
DTM	dermatophyte transport medium	PTT	partial thromboplastin time
		RBC	red blood cell
ELISA	enzyme-linked immunofluorescent assay	(r)RNA	(ribosomal) ribonucleic acid
		RT-PCR	reverse transcription polymerase chain reaction
EPO	erythropoietin		
FCV	feline calicivirus	SC	subcutaneous
FCoV	feline coronavirus	SLE	systemic lupus erythematosus
FDP	fibrin degradation product	SPA	*Staphylococcus* protein A
FeLV	feline leukemia virus	TNR	trap–neuter–return (program)
FeSV	feline sarcoma virus	TPN	total parenteral nutrition
FHV	feline herpesvirus	UMN	upper motor neuron
FIP	feline infectious peritonitis	UPC	urine protein to creatinine ratio
FIV	feline immunodeficiency virus		
FPV	feline panleukopenia virus/feline parvovirus	UTI	urinary tract infection
		VS-FCV	virulent strain feline calicivirus
FUO	fever of unknown origin		
G-CSF	human recombinant granulocyte colony-stimulation factor	WBC	white blood cell

1 A 4-year-old castrated male domestic shorthair cat was seen because of a 7-day history of rigidity of the left thoracic limb (1). Sometimes, episodes of severe muscle spasm were superimposed. Forelimb rigidity had developed over a 72-hour period, but was subsequently nonprogressive. Otherwise, the cat had seemed quite well. It was eating and drinking normally, and could move

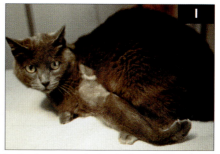

around the house. Apart from the affected limb, the general physical and neurologic examinations were unremarkable. There was a small scab below the left elbow. The limb had markedly increased muscle tone and an increased triceps reflex, and there was normal sensation in the left front paw.

i. What are the differential diagnoses?
ii. What additional evaluation is indicated?
iii. Are radiographs of the spine and a myelogram likely to be helpful in this situation?
iv. Are electrodiagnostic studies likely to be useful?

2 A 2-year-old castrated male domestic shorthaired cat (2) was seen because of acute vomiting for 3 days. The cat had been obtained from a shelter 1 month previously and lived both indoors and outdoors. At presentation, the only preventative care the cat had received was one vaccination against rabies. Physical examination revealed depression, lethargy, hypersalivation, about 7% dehydration and pain on abdominal palpation. The body temperature was 40.9°C.

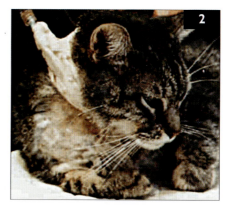

Blood profile	Results
RBC	10.4×10^{12}/l
Platelets	156×10^{9}/l
WBC	0.40×10^{9}/l
Mature neutrophils	0.12×10^{9}/l
Lymphocytes	0.12×10^{9}/l

i. What is the most likely diagnosis in this cat?
ii. What tests should be done next?

1 i. The only likely diagnosis in a cat with this presentation is localized (or local) tetanus.

ii. Local tetanus is a clinical diagnosis, and tetanus is the only infectious disease that is usually diagnosed just based on the clinical findings. In most cases, there is insufficient tetanus toxin present in the circulation for mouse inoculation studies. In early cases it may be possible to culture *Clostridium tetani* from the wound using meticulous anerobic culture techniques. The presence of a wound also lends strong support to a diagnosis of local tetanus, but not all affected animals have a detectable wound. Localized tetanus occurs in cases of minimal toxin elaboration, such that when the toxin is transported retrograde up the peripheral nerves, there is only enough to interfere with inhibitory neurotransmitter release in the motor neuron pools of the affected limb.

iii. Radiographs of the spine and myelography are unlikely to provide any useful diagnostic information in this cat.

iv. Electromyography shows persistent motor unit discharges even under deep anesthesia, confirming the clinical observation of increased activity in motor nerve axons subserving the affected limb, but is usually not necessary to confirm the diagnosis.

2 i. In young animals with inadequate vaccination and worming histories, the most common causes of gastrointestinal disease are: (1) infectious, (2) parasitic, and (3) dietary (food intolerance, ingestion of noxious substances and gastrointestinal foreign bodies).

In this young cat with fever and severe leukopenia, feline panleukopenia virus (FPV) infection is the most likely differential diagnosis. The presence of a fever and leukopenia make inflammatory bowel disease unlikely. A foreign body and peritonitis should also be considered, but peritonitis seems less likely in the absence of an inflammatory leukogram. Extra-gastrointestinal disorders are less likely in a young previously healthy animal and could be ruled out with a serum biochemical panel.

ii. Further tests should include: (1) testing for FPV (fecal antigen test), and (2) fecal examination (flotation, direct smear).

If the FPV antigen test is negative, abdominal imaging studies could be performed. A serum biochemical profile is indicated to rule out metabolic causes of vomiting and to guide fluid therapy. Fecal antigen testing for giardiasis and culture for salmonellosis should be considered. An upper gastrointestinal radiographic contrast study should be considered only if foreign body or mechanical obstruction is strongly suspected. However, this carries a risk of vomiting and aspiration. Biopsy (*via* upper gastrointestinal endoscopy or exploratory laparotomy) should only be considered if the cat does not respond to medical care.

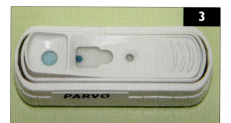

3 Case 3 is the same cat as case 2. A fecal antigen test for parvovirus is negative (3).
i. Does this rule out FPV infection?
ii. What causes feline parvovirosis and how else may it be diagnosed?

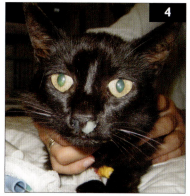

4 A 7-year-old spayed female domestic shorthair cat was seen because of a 3-month history of chronic mucopurulent nasal discharge (4). The cat had received two 10-day courses of antibiotics (amoxicillin and enrofloxacin). During antibiotic treatment nasal discharge became less severe, but it relapsed afterwards. A sample of the nasal discharge had been submitted for bacterial culture and sensitivity testing, and heavy growth of *Pasteurella multocida* was found. Sensitivity testing indicated resistance to amoxicillin and cephalexin. The cat lived indoors, and vaccines were current. Besides the clinical signs related to the nose, the cat was unremarkable. Physical examination revealed purulent nasal discharge from both nares, a slight inspiratory nasal stridor, and slightly enlarged mandibular lymph nodes.
i. What is the most likely reason for nasal discharge?
ii. How useful is a bacterial culture of nasal discharge?
iii. What further tests could be performed?
iv. What are the possible treatment options?

3 i. A negative fecal antigen test result does not rule out FPV infection. Viral shedding is brief and intermittent, and negative results may occur if the test is performed after more than 5–7 days of illness. Viremia occurs before fecal shedding, but negative results are also possible if fecal antigen tests are performed early during clinical illness (e.g. before the onset of diarrhea). Also, positive results are possible following MLV vaccination in healthy animals.

ii. Cats may be infected by FPV or canine parvoviruses (CPV-2a and CPV-2b). Both may cause clinical signs of panleukopenia. Kits that test for fecal canine parvovirus antigen may detect both wild and vaccine strains of both viruses. PCR testing of blood or bone marrow during early infection (viremic phase) may be positive for FPV prior to fecal antigen tests. Parvoviral infection may also be diagnosed *via* fecal electron microscopy, virus isolation, or immunofluorescence staining. Histopathologic examination and immunofluorescence testing are usually carried out in animals that have died. Intestinal biopsies are rarely obtained in acute parvoviral gastroenteritis, as cats are not stable enough to undergo biopsy initially, and later recover with supportive care. Antibody tests are usually negative when the animals are presented, due to the short incubation period. In this case, parvovirus infection was diagnosed by electron microscopy. The cat was treated symptomatically and recovered within a week.

4 i. Diseases that have to be considered are: (1) neoplasia, (2) lymphoplasmacytic rhinitis, (3) trauma, (4) foreign body, (5) dental problems, (6) nasopharyngeal polyps, (7) infectious diseases (e.g. FHV, FCV, cryptococcosis, aspergillosis), and (8) secondary bacterial infections.

ii. Bacterial cultures of nasal discharge are not helpful in establishing a diagnosis. Multiple bacterial organisms can be cultured from the nose of healthy cats; these usually cause secondary infection in chronic nasal diseases. To treat the problem successfully, diagnosis and treatment of the underlying primary disease should be attempted.

iii. The oral cavity should be examined for signs of dental disease, masses deviating the hard or soft palate, or polyps protruding into the nasopharynx. A complete blood count, biochemistry profile, and urinalysis should be performed to detect systemic disease causing immunosuppression or organ dysfunction. Nasal cytology could be performed to look for *Cryptococcus* spp., and a cryptococcal antigen titer could be obtained. To localize the disease process, involvement of the lower airways and sinuses should be investigated. CT or radiographs of the nasal cavity and paranasal sinuses should be followed by rhinoscopy to visualize the disease process and to obtain biopsy samples for histopathology and fungal culture.

iv. Firstly, the underlying disease process should be addressed. If this problem can be treated, secondary bacterial infection should resolve with a broad-spectrum antibiotic given for 2–3 weeks. If the underlying problem cannot be treated successfully, antibiotic pulse therapy or long-term treatment with an antibiotic may be helpful.

5 A 3-year-old spayed female domestic shorthair cat was seen because of scratching her ears and shaking her head. On physical examination, brown crusty debris was seen in both ears (5a). There were excoriations of the skin behind one ear and miliary dermatitis in the dorsal lumbosacral area, as

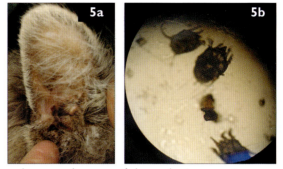

well as extensive excoriation on the ventral aspect of the neck. An organism was seen on microscopic examination (5b).

i. What is the organism shown in the image?
ii. How is it transmitted?
iii. Is this organism specific to cats?
iv. How should the cat be treated?
v. Is the miliary dermatitis related to this organism?

6 A 7-year-old spayed female domestic shorthair cat was seen because of an acute onset of left-sided head tilt and Horner's syndrome (6) 5 days ago. The cat lived indoors and outdoors. It had been vaccinated against FPV, FHV and FCV. It had a lifelong history of chronic nasal discharge and was treated intermittently with antibiotics; the last treatment was 6 months previously. On examination, there was mucopurulent

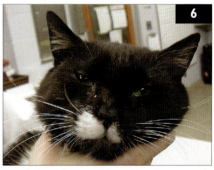

nasal discharge, and the cat showed open-mouth breathing. The external ear canals and the tympanic membranes were normal. The neurologic examination showed head tilt to the left and intermittent falling to the right side on turns and when shaking the head. There was horizontal nystagmus with the fast phase to the right which did not change direction with different positions of the head. Postural reactions, spinal reflexes, and cranial nerves were all normal except for Horner's syndrome of the left eye.

i. What is the neuroanatomic localization?
ii. What are the most likely differential diagnoses?
iii. What further diagnostic steps are suggested?

5 i. The organism is *Otodectes cynotis*, the most common mite to infest the cat.
ii. It is transmitted by direct contact between animals, especially during the neonatal period of the cat. High morbidity is expected in a multiple-cat setting.
iii. Host specificity is not exclusive. This organism can also cause otitis externa in dogs, foxes, and ferrets, and, in people, a pruritic rash on the arms and thorax.
iv. Successful treatment requires treating ears as well as the coat and tail to eliminate a source of reinfestation. The ears should be thoroughly cleaned by removing all of the debris, before treating with a topical miticidal preparation. Topical selemectin, imidicloprid, ivermectin, or fipronil may be used. The cat should also be treated with a flea spray labeled for use on cats. All other cats and possible carriers in the household should also be treated as they may be inapparent carriers. Secondary bacterial infection or inflammation related to a hypersensitivity response may need treatment with a topical antibiotic–corticosteroid combination.
v. Most infestations are limited to the head and neck. Occasionally, generalized infestation may occur. Differential diagnoses for the concurrent miliary skin condition include allergic skin diseases (flea, inhalant, food), other ectoparasites, dermatophytosis, demodicosis, and pyoderma.

6 i. Head tilt is a sign of vestibular disease. Vestibular disease can be either of peripheral or of central origin. Decreased postural reactions, vertical nystagmus or nystagmus which changes direction with different positions of the head or cranial nerve deficits other than facial paresis or Horner's syndrome are indicative of central vestibular disease. Head tilt and falling are usually ipsilateral to the lesion, and the fast phase of the nystagmus usually points away from it. Paradoxical vestibular disease with head tilt and fast phase of the nystagmus towards the side of the lesion may occur with some types of central vestibular disease. In this cat, the neurologic examination indicated peripheral vestibular disease (inner ear, CN VIII). Horner's syndrome can result from a variety of lesions in the sympathetic pathway (diencephalon, brainstem, spinal cord, T1–T3 nerve roots, thorax, vagosympathetic trunk, middle ear or orbit). Middle ear disease is the most likely cause of Horner's syndrome in this cat.
ii. Inflammatory, idiopathic, and neoplastic diseases are the most frequent causes of peripheral vestibular disease in cats. Toxic and vascular causes, anomaly, and trauma are rare. Otitis media is a common consequence of upper respiratory tract disease in cats. Normal findings on otoscopic examination cannot exclude otitis media. Horner's syndrome is a frequent sign of otitis media in cats.
iii. Imaging of the tympanic bullae with MRI or CT should be performed. Alternatively, radiographic assessment of the tympanic bulla can be done. Myringotomy may be tried to obtain a specimen for cytology and bacterial culture.

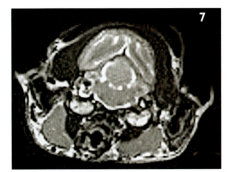

7 Case 7 is the same cat as case 6. Transverse MR images (T2) showed that both bullae were filled with tissue and fluid. Additional views showed complete loss of nasal turbinates (7 [courtesy of Prof. U. Matis, LMU University of Munich]).
i. What treatment options can be suggested?
ii. What are the risks involved with the treatment?

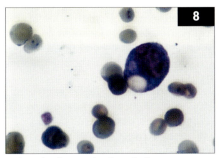

8 A 4-year-old castrated male domestic shorthair cat was seen because of a 3-day history of being less energetic than normal. On physical examination, the cat was alert but less assertive than expected. Its oral mucous membranes were pale and slightly icteric. Abdominal palpation revealed splenomegaly, which was confirmed radiographically. The complete blood count revealed a macrocytic, hypochromic anemia (hematocrit 0.16 l/l) with only few reticulocytes (5×10^9/l) present. A blood smear was examined (8).
i. What are the clinically significant abnormalities seen in the blood smear?
ii. What are the clinically relevant differences between these organisms?
iii. How do cats become infected with these organisms?
iv. How is this disease treated?
v. What is the prognosis?

7 i. Chronic otitis media/interna is often managed surgically with ventral bulla osteotomy. Ventral osteotomy is also needed for removal of inflammatory polyps. Otitis media/interna may also be treated conservatively with antibiotics or antifungals as indicated by culture and cytology results. Amoxicillin/clavulanate (22 mg/kg bid) combined with clindamycin or metronidazole can be used until culture results are available. Topical treatment alone is insufficient and long-term (>8 weeks) parenteral treatment is required. Myringotomy should be considered if the tympanic membrane appears bulged or chronically inflamed. Saline flushing of the middle ear for treatment of exudative otitis media in cats is considered less effective than in dogs because of the two compartments of the tympanic cavity in this species.

ii. Horner's syndrome, facial paresis, inner ear and hypoglossal nerve damage can occur secondary to surgery. Facial paresis may be associated with keratoconjunctivitis sicca because of loss of parasympathetic innervation of the lacrimal glands. Vestibular signs may also be slightly more pronounced following anesthesia due to loss of central compensatory mechanisms.

8 i. *Mycoplasma* organisms are seen on the surface of the red cells. *Mycoplasma haemofelis* and *M. haemominutum* are the two most common hemotrophic *Mycoplasma* spp. of cats. An additional species has been identified recently in Switzerland (candidatus *M. turicensis*). Hemotrophic *Mycoplasma* spp. attach to red blood cells, causing alteration of the cell membrane. Parasitized erythrocytes are cleared from circulation by the spleen leaving normal, nonparasitized red blood cells in circulation. Thus, depending on when the blood sample is collected, infected cells may or may not be apparent.

ii. *M. haemofelis* is more likely to cause clinical disease (anemia); *M. haemominutum* infections are usually inapparent. Morphology cannot be relied on to differentiate between them; PCR is required for specific identification.

iii. Fleas and possibly other blood-sucking arthropods are the primary means of transmission; neonatal kittens may be infected.

iv. Doxycycline and enrofloxacin are the drugs of choice. Several cautions must be observed: because doxycycline can cause esophageal strictures, suspensions should be used, or water should be administered after using a tablet or capsule. Cats with severe anemia may benefit from glucocorticoids (prednisolone 1–2 mg/kg PO q 12 hrs) concurrently to reduce splenic erythrophagocytosis and suppress secondary immune-mediated autoimmune hemolytic anemia. This dose may be tapered as the hematocrit increases. In life-threatening anemia, blood transfusions should be administered.

v. Despite successful clinical remission following antimicrobial therapy, most cats remain inapparent carriers.

9 A 4-year-old castra-ted male domestic longhair cat was seen because of a swollen tongue, making it unable to close its mouth (**9a**). It lived in an animal shelter. On physical examination, it was febrile and had

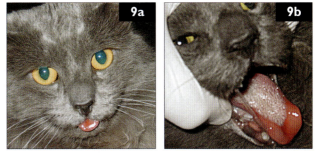

an extensive horseshoe-shaped lingual ulcer (**9b**). There were 56 other cats in the ward, all housed individually. Cages were cleaned daily with a quaternary ammonium disinfectant, diluted with an unmeasured amount of water. All were vaccinated on intake with SC and intranasal vaccines against FPV, FHV, and FCV; all were examined now. Six additional affected cats were discovered; all were adults. The affected cats were isolated. The following day, another six cats were showing similar signs.
i. What are the most likely causes of this outbreak?
ii. What steps should be taken to control the problem and protect the shelter cats while awaiting a definitive diagnosis?

10 A 2-year-old intact female dom-estic shorthair cat was seen because of rapidly progressive dyspnea over the previous 3 days. The cat had been imported from Spain to Florida a year earlier. It was kept primarily indoors with limited outside access. Vaccin-ations against FPV, FHV, FCV, and rabies were current. On physical examination, the cat was overtly

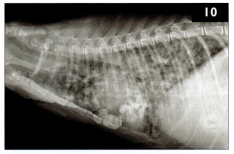

dyspneic with open-mouth breathing. Body temperature (40.2°C), heart rate (220 bpm), and respiratory rate (65 bpm) were all increased. Harsh lung sounds were auscultated in all lung fields. Mild cranial abdominal organomegaly was palpated. The rest of the physical examination was unremarkable. Thoracic radiographs were obtained when the cat was stabilized (**10**).
i. What is the first priority for treatment of this cat?
ii. What is the radiographic interpretation?
iii. What are the differential diagnoses?
iv. What should be done to make a diagnosis?

9, 10: Answers

9 i. The two most likely causes are FCV infection and disinfectant toxicity. Quaternary ammonium compounds do not reliably inactivate FCV. The frequency of oral ulceration, and the fact that long-term residents were more frequently affected than newer residents, suggests disinfectant toxicity may be more likely than FCV infection. Staff should be closely questioned and observed regarding disinfectant use, and samples of all disinfectants in use collected. Oropharyngeal swabs should be obtained from all cats; however, false positive FCV results may occur because of recent vaccination with an MLV vaccine. If most or all cats are negative for FCV, this can be ruled out.

ii. All affected cats should be moved into an isolation area and handled carefully until FCV has been ruled out. They should be treated with analgesics and broad-spectrum antibiotics to control secondary bacterial infections. Chlorhexidine mouth rinses may also be helpful. If disinfectant toxicity is strongly suspected, exposed cats should be bathed in warm water and mild detergent. Movement of cats should be halted until a diagnosis is reached. Cages should be cleaned with mild detergent followed by disinfection with a product with action against FCV. Shelter and veterinary staff should be taught about using disinfectants at the correct dilution. In this case, an open spray bottle of disinfectant, missing its top, was seen on a counter.

10 i. The first priority is to stabilize the cat's condition. It was immediately placed in an oxygen cage containing 60% oxygen. Acute respiratory distress in cats is often due to congestive heart failure, and a heart murmur is not always present. Acute bronchial asthma or an airway foreign body can also cause life-threatening respiratory distress. However, none of these conditions are typically associated with fever. The ability to auscultate lung sounds in all fields argued against pleural effusion or pneumothorax. Bronchodilator therapy was initiated with terbutaline, and the cat was rested in oxygen.

ii. Thoracic radiographs revealed a severe diffuse multifocal nodular interstitial infiltrate obscuring the cardiac silhouette. Some of the nodules appeared to be mineralized.

iii. The primary differential diagnoses for this radiographic pattern in a febrile cat include fungal, mycobacterial, protozoal, and neoplastic conditions. Because the cat is very young, infectious causes are thought to be more likely than a neoplasm.

iv. A complete blood count, biochemisty panel, urinalysis, and feline leukemia virus (FeLV) and feline immunodeficiency virus (FIV) tests should be performed to evaluate for inflammatory responses, systemic disease, and possible immunosuppressive conditions. Since the disease is diffuse, a fine-needle aspirate of the lung could be performed with minimal stress and without the risk of anesthesia. The primary risks of such a procedure would be creation of a pneumothorax or pulmonary hemorrhage.

11 Case **11** is the same cat as case **10**.

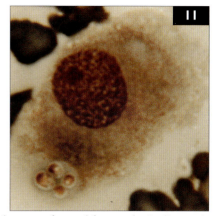

Blood profile/ biochemistry panel	Results
Hematocrit – mild nonregenerative anemia	0.26 l/l
Neutrophilia	23.5×10^9/l
Left shift band neutrophils	2.3×10^9/l
ALT – mild increase	198 IU/l
Hypoalbuminemia	22 g/l
Hyperglobulinemia	68 g/l

FeLV and FIV tests were negative. A fine-needle aspirate of the caudodorsal lung field was performed for cytologic diagnosis (**11**).
i. What is the diagnosis?
ii. Was the disease likely acquired in Spain or in Florida?
iii. What is the treatment?
iv. What is the prognosis?

12 A 9-year-old intact female Norwegian Forest Cat (**12**) was seen for an annual routine examination and consultation. The cat came from a household with 12 adult cats. Two months ago, one adult cat in the household developed feline infectious peritonitis (FIP) and was euthanized. All of the cats were kept strictly indoors in a 120 m² apartment, and all cats had contact with each other. This cat had been used for breeding several years ago but had not had a litter

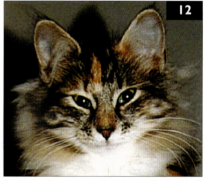

in the last 3 years. The cat had been healthy since the last annual visit, and physical examination was unremarkable.
i. How high is the risk that this cat will also develop FIP?
ii. What can be done to reduce the risk of FIP in this household?
iii. Does early weaning help?
iv. What are the recommendations for a breeding facility?

11 i. Four yeast-like organisms are contained within the cytoplasm of a macrophage recovered by fine-needle aspiration of the lung. The organisms are most consistent with *Histoplasma capsulatum*. The radiographic findings of diffuse miliary to nodular interstitial infiltrates with mineralization are classic findings in feline histoplasmosis.

ii. The infection was most likely acquired in Florida as it has not been diagnosed in Europe.

iii. Treatment was initiated with itraconazole (10 mg/kg PO q 12 h) and intravenous fluids at a maintenance rate. The cat was maintained in the oxygen cage, but its condition deteriorated. Dexamethasone (0.2 mg/kg SC q 12 h) was administered for 3 days to combat suspected increased pulmonary inflammation secondary to treatment-induced fungal death. The condition stabilized and then gradually improved to the point that oxygen supplementation was withdrawn on day 7. By day 14, the cat was maintaining hydration and eating. It was discharged with itraconazole.

iv. For cats that survive the initial crisis, the prognosis for recovery is good. Like most other systemic fungal infections, antifungal therapy is generally required for many months and should be continued until there has been no evidence of infection by clinicopathological tests or radiography for at least 1–2 months. This cat made a complete recovery, and itraconazole was discontinued after 9 months of therapy.

12 i. The risk to develop FIP in a multi-cat household in which FCoV is endemic is 5–10%. It is higher if the cat is less than 6 months old, or immunosuppressed; it also depends on the virulence of the FCoV strain.

ii. Households of less than five cats can spontaneously become FCoV-free, but probably not those with more than ten cats. Reducing the number of cats (especially those <12 months old) and frequent cleaning of the litter boxes and surfaces can minimize loads. Antibody testing and segregation can reduce exposure. Alternatively, PCR testing can be performed to detect persistent shedders. In multiple-cat environments, 40–60% of cats shed virus in their feces at any given time. If cats remain PCR-positive for more than 6 weeks, they should be removed.

iii. Kittens of FCoV-shedding queens are protected from infection by maternally-derived antibodies until they are 5–6 weeks old. An early-weaning protocol to prevent FCoV infection in kittens has been proposed. If early weaning is done correctly and combined with strict hygiene, it might help to prevent FCoV infection in these kittens.

iv. It may be possible to maximize heritable resistance to FIP in breeding catteries. Genetically susceptible cats are approximately twice as likely to develop FIP than other cats. If a cat has two or more litters in which kittens develop FIP, she should not be bred from again.

13 An adult (age unknown) female (neutering history unknown) domestic shorthair cat in an animal shelter was found dead in its cage with edematous ulcerated feet (**13a**). This shelter was a large municipal shelter. Trapped feral cats are housed in a room separate from the rest of the feline shelter population. The cages were standard steel but had slatted floors. Throughout the day, several cats died with the same changes. Further inspection also found live cats with similar lesions of varying severity and others with swollen, distorted faces (**13b**). Staff reported that this had been an ongoing problem for the last 4 months.

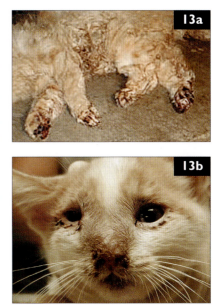

i. What are the primary rule-outs for this problem?

ii. What further information is needed to investigate this outbreak?

14 Case **14** is the same cat as in case **13**. Necropsies of several of the dead cats revealed suppurative and necrotizing rhinitis and frontal sinusitis in several cats. There was also evidence of suppurative meningitis, with extensive regions of submeningeal pus overlying the cerebral cortices. The distal limbs and paws showed regions of ulceration with edema (**14a**), hemorrhage, and necrosis (**14b**). Microbiological culture was performed on samples from several pathological lesions. Gram-positive nonmotile facultatively anerobic b-hemolytic cocci were isolated.

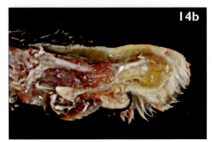
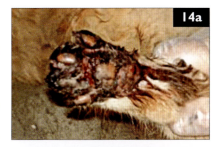

i. What is the diagnosis?

ii. What are predisposing factors that may lead to this disease?

iii. What advice should be given to this shelter to handle this outbreak?

13 i. An infectious etiology is likely considering the history, number of affected cats, location, and population of animals involved. Primary rule-outs include viral or bacterial causes.

ii. A thorough visual inspection of the facility is needed as these cats have unknown histories and they are not amenable to routine physical examinations or tests. This includes examining intake protocols, the cages, cage supplies (e.g. litter boxes, bowls, towels), and the room in general. It is also important to determine how the staff clean and what types of cleaners and disinfectants are used. It is often best to observe staff as they perform their routine with these animals. Most importantly, necropsy is invaluable when investigating outbreaks in shelters.

14 i. The history, clinical signs and microbiology indicate infection with *Streptococcus canis* possessing the Lancefield group G antigen. These are commensal microflora of cats; however, severe infections can occur, usually in kittens but also in older cats in shelter-type conditions.

ii. Neonatal kittens can succumb to generalized *S. canis* septicemia and older juveniles to cervical lymphadenitis. In outbreaks, disease can also be seen in adult cats. These cases are generally opportunistic and result from wounds, trauma, surgical procedures, viral infections, and/or immunosuppressive conditions. Feral cats in shelters are very stressed due to their captivity and confinement. The cats here also have potentially paw-damaging cage floors.

iii. In shelter medicine, it is paramount to consider the well-being of the entire shelter's cat population. Therefore, all affected cats were euthanized to prevent further suffering and disease transmission. In addition, there is a low zoonotic potential from *S. canis* to humans. Unaffected cats should be moved to another room into new cages with solid floors. All empty cages that are to be reused must be completely cleaned and then disinfected with bleach. Steam cleaning, mechanical brushing, proper contact time with an adequate disinfectant, and complete drying are mandatory. It is possible to treat *Streptococcus* spp. infections with various penicillins if isolation facilities are available for the treatment period.

15 Case 15 is the same as cases 13 and 14. The shelter proceeded to follow the above recommendations and reported no new cases for several weeks when the outbreak began to repeat itself. On interviewing the staff, it was found out that feral cats were initially removed from traps and placed into cages with the use of a rabies pole (15a).

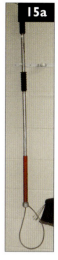

i. What should be investigated this time?
ii. What should the shelter staff be asked?

16 A 4-year-old spayed female domestic shorthair cat (16a) was seen because of weight loss despite a good appetite until 2 weeks prior to presentation when it stopped eating well. The cat lived primarily outdoors, and was last vaccinated against FPV, FHV, FCV, and rabies at 1 year old. It was the owners' only cat; it weighed only 3 kg. On abdominal palpation, both kidneys were very irregular (16b) and were enlarged. The abdominal radiograph (16c) confirmed bilateral renomegaly. A CBC showed that the cat had a mild nonregenerative anemia; a biochemistry panel revealed elevations of creatinine (230 mmol/l) and urea (15 mmol/l); and a urinalysis was normal, with an SG of 1.046. The cat was treated with lactated Ringer's initially. After this, the urea and creatinine concentrations were still elevated, and the urine specific gravity was 1.022.

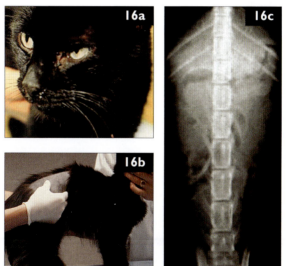

i. What are the cat's problems?
ii. What are the differential diagnoses?
iii. What is an appropriate further diagnostic plan?

15 i. All focus had been on the cats in the cages. The re-emergence of disease now requires looking at other sources of infection or trauma.

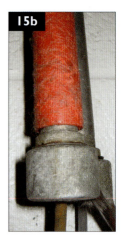

ii. Discussions with staff revealed that the pole used to remove feral cats from traps and place them into cages was the same pole that was also used to remove cats from cages for transport and euthanasia. The pole was examined and found to be covered in hair and had evidence of copious bite marks along the sponge-covered handle (**15b**). It was obvious that the cats were being injured during movement and that the pole could not be appropriately cleaned. The pole was removed and the cats were subsequently transferred from cage to carrier and *vice versa* by juxtaposing the doors and allowing the cats to move on their own. The *Streptococcus canis* outbreaks were thus stopped.

16 i. The presenting problem is weight loss associated with a poor appetite. Renomegaly is the predominant physical abnormality, and there is mild azotemia.

ii. Azotemia can be prerenal, renal, or postrenal.

The cat is only mildly azotemic, so this does not explain the partial anorexia and weight loss. There is no evidence for prerenal or postrenal azotemia. Concentrated urine does not necessarily exclude renal disease as the cause of azotemia in cats. Here, the renomegaly suggests this. Diseases that can result in bilateral renomegaly in cats include lymphoma, polycystic renal disease, granulomatous nephritis (e.g. with FIP), renal amyloidosis, and hydronephrosis.

iii. The diagnostic plan should include testing for FeLV (and FIV). Renal ultrasonography should be performed; ultrasonic imaging of the kidneys is useful to diagnose polycystic disease and hydronephrosis. If the kidneys are solid, a renal aspirate should be performed; this may diagnose renal lymphoma. If this is nondiagnostic, a renal biopsy is indicated; this is necessary to diagnose granulomatous nephritis and amyloidosis. Infection with FeLV is associated with renal lymphoma in some cats, and so an FeLV (and FIV) test is indicated in the predominately outdoor cat. Infection with FeLV can also result in a nonregenerative anemia with a mildly increased MCV. The cat was diagnosed with renal lymphoma based on the aspirate cytology (**16d**), and tested positive for FeLV.

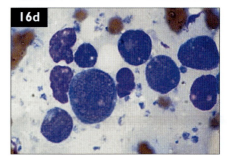

17 Five 8-week-old kittens from a local rescue group were admitted for routine ovariohysterectomy/castration. They were boarded in an isolation area at the clinic. All areas were routinely cleaned with a quaternary ammonium disinfectant. Within 3 days of surgery, all members of the litter became febrile (body temperatures 39.0–40.5°C) and developed oral ulceration, serous nasal and ocular discharge and sneezing. Four adult blood-donor cats were kept in an adjacent ward. They had been vaccinated 18 months previously against FPV, FHV, and FCV. Within 3 days of the kittens showing clinical signs, three of them developed multiple lingual and palatal ulcers (17a), alopecia, skin ulceration, oozing of many skin areas (17b), edema, and mild increases of body temperature.

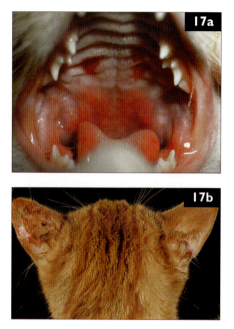

i. What are the most likely differential diagnoses?
ii. What diagnostic tests could be used to determine the cause?
iii. What steps should be taken to protect clients' pets while awaiting a diagnosis?

18 A 7-year-old castrated male Burmese cat was seen because of a history of chronic coughing that had responded in the past to treatment with corticosteroids. It was presented in acute respiratory distress with bilateral purulent nasal discharge. Thoracic radiographs showed a marked bronchial pattern, flattening of the diaphragm, and consolidation of the caudal part of the left cranial lung lobe. Air bronchograms were visible within the consolidated lung lobe. A cytologic preparation of bronchoalveolar lavage (BAL) was prepared (18) (modified Wrights–Giemsa).

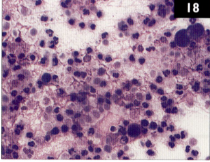

i. What are the differential diagnoses based on the radiographic findings?
ii. What does the cytology show?

17 i. FCV infection is the most likely cause. This may occur in vaccinated cats. Virulent systemic FCV strains (VS-FCV) associated with edema (**17c**), widespread alopecia, ulceration, and death have been reported. This case had many features of VS-FCV. Disinfectant toxicity (quaternary ammonium or phenol) should also be considered; this can cause oral and skin ulceration, fever, upper and lower respiratory disease, and death in cats.

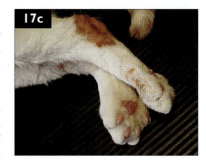

ii. Oropharyngeal swabs and serum from affected cats should be submitted for viral culture or PCR for FCV. Subclinical carriage is common; therefore, positive results from oropharyngeal swabs do not prove disease. A positive result from blood is more suggestive, as circulating virus is only present during acute disease. However, blood is commonly negative, even in acutely infected cats. Definitive diagnosis of VS-FCV can only be made *via* necropsy and demonstration of characteristic lesions and presence of virus in tissues. A diagnosis of disinfectant toxicity is made by ruling out other causes, coupled with resolution of disease following its removal.

iii. All affected cats should be isolated. Access should be restricted to limited staff members, and full protective clothing worn. Separate equipment should be used for cleaning and care. All asymptomatic but exposed cats should also be strictly isolated: they may be carriers. Use of the quaternary ammonium disinfectant should be discontinued until toxicity has been ruled out.

18 i. The radiographic findings are suggestive of chronic inflammatory airway disease (e.g. asthma). Consolidation of the right middle-lung lobe and flattening of the diaphragm are common radiographic signs of chronic inflammatory airway disease. In this case consolidation of the left cranial lung lobe and purulent nasal discharge most likely indicate a secondary bronchopneumonia. Concurrent viral upper respiratory disease or *Mycoplasma* spp. infection could cause nasal discharge. *Mycoplasma* spp. may cause upper and lower respiratory tract infections in cats. Differential diagnoses include primary pneumonia (e.g. aspiration pneumonia), respiratory parasitism, heartworm infection, or neoplasia.

ii. There is a thick background of mucus and lysed cells on the BAL preparation. Large numbers of intact inflammatory cells are present. These are neutrophils predominantly, with lower numbers of lymphocytes, macrophages, and dark-staining ciliated epithelial cells. No bacteria can be seen. This does not rule out the presence of *Mycoplasma* spp. which, due to their lack of a rigid cell wall, are not detected on routine stains.

19 Case **19** is the same cat as case **18**. Culture of the BAL yielded a pure growth of a *Mycoplasma* spp. (**19**).
i. What is the significance of isolating a pure growth of a *Mycoplasma* spp. from a BAL in a cat?
ii. How should this cat be treated?

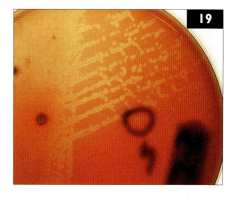

20 A 3-year-old spayed female domestic longhair cat was seen because of poor appetite and weight loss. It was vaccinated against FPV, FHV, FCV, FeLV, and rabies, and was on heartworm preventive. It was the only cat in the household. The distal left front leg was mildly swollen (**20a**), but the swelling was not hot. A complete blood count, biochemistry panel, and urinalysis were performed. The abnormal results were:

Blood profile/biochemistry panel	Results
Mature neutrophils	12.25×10^9/l
Lymphocytes	1.0×10^9/l
Total protein	50 g/l
Albumin	11 g/l
Calcium	1.9 mmol/l
Urinalysis	
Protein	++++
Specific gravity	1.024

i. What are the cat's problems?
ii. What are the differential diagnoses?
iii. What is an appropriate further diagnostic plan?
iv. Should any therapy be considered pending further diagnostic testing?

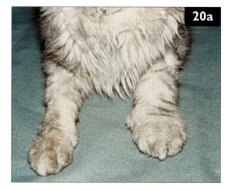

19 i. *Mycoplasma* spp. are not present in the lower airways of healthy cats. However, they have been isolated from BAL of up to 25% of cats with lower airway disease. *Mycoplasma* spp. may cause significant structural damage to airway epithelium. In people, *M. pneumoniae* infection causes airway hyper-reactivity and is known to trigger or exacerbate asthma attacks. In this cat, it is likely that its chronic inflammatory airway disease resulted in compromise of respiratory defense mechanisms and secondary mycoplasmal pneumonia.
ii. Antibiotic susceptibility testing is not routinely available for feline mycoplasmal isolates. *Mycoplasma* spp. are usually susceptible to macrolides, azalides, tetra-cyclines, chloramphenicol, fluoroquinolones, clindamycin, and aminoglycosides. Therapy should be given for a minimum of 4 weeks. The cat's chronic airway disease should be treated with an inhaled corticosteroid, such as fluticasone and a bronchodilator such as salbutamol in addition. These may be administered to the cat using a metered-dose inhaler.

20 i. There is a marked hypoalbuminemia associated with a marked proteinuria. Although the cat is not azotemic, the urine specific gravity is low in comparison to the highly concentrated urine typical of young cats. Protein-losing nephropathy can explain the findings.
ii. Protein-losing nephropathies in cats are due to glomerulopathy, caused by renal amyloidosis or glomerulonephritis. Glomerulonephritis is the most common cause in cats; renal amyloidosis is rare. Glomerulonephritis has many causes, but usually no cause is determined.
iii. The diagnostic plan should include testing for FeLV and FIV and measurement of the urine protein to creatinine ratio. The systolic blood pressure should also be measured to rule out hypertension. If tests for infectious diseases are negative, thoracic and abdominal radiographs and abdominal ultrasound are indicated to evaluate for an underlying inflammatory or neoplastic disease. If these tests are negative, a renal biopsy is indicated. Biopsy confirmed glomerulonephritis in this cat (**20b**), but no infectious cause could be identified.
iv. Pending test results, symptomatic therapy should be instituted. This consists of the gradual introduction of a diet designed for feline renal failure. However, overzealous protein restriction should be avoided. In addition, the administration of an ACE inhibitor (e.g. benazepril) may reduce the severity of the proteinuria and may improve the prognosis.

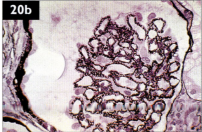

20b

21 A 10-year-old castrated male domestic shorthair cat was seen because of chronic vomiting, inappetence and weight loss of 6 months' duration. Metronidazole had been given, but wasn't helpful. The cat lived indoors and outdoors, received heartworm preventative, and was current on vaccinations against FPV, FHV, FCV, FeLV, FCoV,

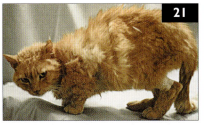

and rabies. Physical examination showed a very thin body condition and an unkempt haircoat (21). A complete blood count, biochemical panel, T4 test, and urinalysis were normal except for a slight hypoalbuminemia. Three fecal flotations were negative for parasitic ova and *Giardia* spp. Tests for FeLV and FIV, and abdominal imaging studies, were normal. Endoscopic examination revealed gastritis with prominent lymphoid follicles, pinpoint mucosal hemorrhages, and duodenitis. Intestinal biopsies revealed moderate to severe lymphocytic–plasmacytic inflammation. Special stains showed many *Helicobacter* spp. bacteria within gastric glands.
i. How should this cat be treated?
ii. How should this cat be monitored?

22 A 7-year-old castrated male domestic shorthair cat was seen because it had developed a small subcutaneous mass on the left flank 8 months earlier. After initial unsuccessful antibiotic therapy, the mass had been surgically removed. A few months later, the lesion had returned and started to spread. The cat was an indoor/outdoor cat living in a multi-cat household. On physical examination, the cat was bright and alert. The skin lesions consisted of alopecia with multiple circular, deep and draining skin ulcers of variable size on the left flank (22a) extending to the caudodorsal area (22b). Two soft subcutaneous masses were also palpated in the inguinal area.

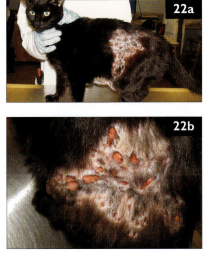

i. List the three most likely differential diagnoses for this type of skin lesion.
ii. What dermatologic tests should be performed?
iii. Which of the differential diagnoses produce tissue granules?
iv. If an acid-fast stained tissue section shows partially acid-fast filamentous organisms, what is the tentative diagnosis?

21 i. The question is whether this cat's gastrointestinal lesions are due to *Helicobacter* spp. infection, or whether other underlying gastrointestinal disease (e.g. inflammatory bowel disease [IBD], food sensitivity) is present. It would be prudent to change the cat's food to a hypoallergenic diet to minimize mucosal inflammation. Treatment for *Helicobacter* spp. consists of combination drug therapy (antibiotics with an antisecretory drug) for 2–4 weeks. Optimal drug combinations and durations of treatment are unknown for cats. If clinical signs do not improve, or if they relapse following cessation, further treatment for IBD may be indicated.

ii. As noninvasive tests for *Helicobacter* spp. in cats are not currently available, repeat gastroduodenoscopy should ideally be performed at the conclusion of treatment to determine whether *Helicobacter* spp. has been eradicated and to reassess gastrointestinal morphologic changes. Resolution of clinical signs, apparent eradication of the organism, and gross and histologic resolution of gastrointestinal inflammation would suggest the cat's disease was indeed due to the presence of *Helicobacter* spp. If repeat gastroduodenoscopy is not an option, the cat should be monitored by following clinical signs, body weight, body condition, and serum albumin concentration. PCR testing for *Helicobacter* spp. in fecal samples may be available in the future, allowing less invasive testing.

22 i. The three most likely differential diagnoses are nocardiosis, mycobacteriosis, and actinomycosis. These three conditions are clinically indistinguishable and are characterized by nodular to diffuse cellulitis, draining tracts, ulcerated nodules, and abscesses with fistulation most commonly located on limbs, feet, or ventral abdomen. Respiratory signs, fever, anorexia, depression, and lymphadenopathy may be present as well.

ii. Cytology, bacterial culture, and histopathology should be performed. Cytology from exudates or fine-needle aspirates shows pyogranulomatous inflammation in these cases. Gram-positive filamentous, beaded to rod-shaped organisms can occasionally be found. They are acid-fast (mycobacteriosis), partially acid-fast (nocardiosis), or non-acid-fast (actinomycosis). Histopathology is consistent with a nodular to diffuse pyogranulomatous dermatitis and panniculitis with intra-lesional tissue granules. In bacterial cultures (aerobic and anerobic), *Actinomyces* spp. require anerobic conditions, whereas *Nocardia* spp. and opportunistic *Mycobacteria* spp. prefer aerobic conditions.

iii. Tissue granules are produced by *Nocardia* spp. and *Actinomyces* spp.

iv. The diagnosis in this cat is nocardiosis. *Actinomyces* spp. do not show acid-fast staining within the tissue granules, whereas mycobacterial organisms are acid-fast positive but do not produce tissue granules. Despite these differences, the diagnosis should be confirmed by culture of the organism.

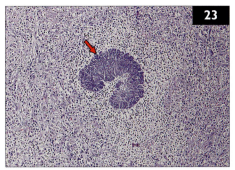

23 Case 23 is the same cat as case 22. Histopathology showed a nodular to diffuse pyogranulomatous dermatitis and panniculitis with intralesional tissue granules (23, arrow) (hematoxylin and eosin [H&E] stain), and *Nocardia* spp. were cultured.
i. Why is isolation of this organism important?
ii. What is the medical management plan?

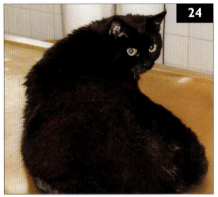

24 A 12-year-old spayed female Persian cat was seen for its annual routine examination. Physical examination revealed a generally sparse coat with crusts and white flakes (24). The cat was noted to scratch itself in the examination room.
i. What are the differential diagnoses for the coat condition?
ii. What diagnostic tests are appropriate to confirm the diagnosis?
iii. Could there be a zoonotic issue?
iv. What is the appropriate treatment?

23 i. Isolation and antimicrobial susceptibility testing of clinical isolates of *Nocardia* spp. are important, because individual strains show differences in their susceptibility pattern. Most *Nocardia* spp. isolates are susceptible to sulfonamides, except for *Nocardia otitidiscaviarum*. *Nocardia nova* is usually sensitive to erythromycin, but *Nocardia farcinia* is not.

ii. A combination of surgical excision or drainage of infected tissue and long-term antibiotic therapy is the treatment of choice. If susceptibility test results are not available, sulfonamides are considered the first-line drug for the treatment of nocardiosis. Clinical improvement should be observed within 10 days after starting treatment, and therapy should be continued for 1 month beyond complete clinical resolution. However, due to the potential risk of side-effects such as myelosuppression during prolonged sulfonamide application, or in the case of lack of response to therapy, alternative treatment options should be considered.

Trimethoprim/sulfonamide (15 mg/kg PO q 12 h) or Amoxicillin/clavulanate (10–20 mg/kg PO q 12 h) or Ampicillin (20–40 mg/kg PO q 12 h)	alone or in combination with	Erythromycin (10–15 mg/kg PO q 8 h) or Clarithromycin (7.5 mg/kg PO q 12 h) or Tetracycline (20 mg/kg PO q 8 h) or Clindamycin (11–24 mg/kg PO q 24 h)

24 i. Cheyletiellosis, demodicosis, dermatophytosis, dry environment, chronic allergic skin disease, and malnutrition are the main differential diagnoses.

ii. Microscopic examination of coat brushings (scale, debris, hair) collected on a piece of paper has a higher diagnostic yield than the 'sticky tape' test alone. A magnifying lens may be adequate for evaluating this. The tape test is performed by applying clear tape to the hair coat of the cat and then placing the tape onto a microscope slide to examine for parasites and eggs attached to the hairs. Mites may occasionally be found on fecal examination of cats who have groomed the mites from their coat.

iii. Cheyletiellosis was diagnosed in this case. This is a zoonotic disease and causes a pruritic rash on the arms and trunk in about 20–30% of human cases.

iv. Topical fipronil should be applied twice, three weeks apart. Selemectin and ivermectin are also effective. As the mites are able to live away from their host for at least 1 month, thorough cleansing of the environment is important. The environment may be a significant reservoir for reinfestation in catteries or uncared-for environments.

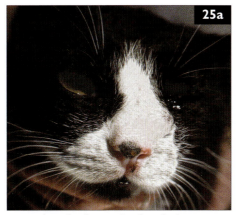

25 A 2-year-old castrated male domestic shorthair cat was seen in Turin, Italy because of a 2-week history of sneezing, mucopurulent bilateral nasal discharge, and nasal swelling. On physical examination, stridor, inspiratory dyspnea, exophthalmus, and oculonasal discharge were present (25a). The cat had been tested FIV-positive previously.
i. What are the main differential diagnoses for the problems?
ii. What diagnostic procedures should be performed?

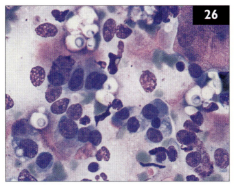

26 Case 26 is the same cat as case 25. A fine-needle aspirate was obtained from the lesion (26) (May–Gruenwald–Giemsa stain).
i. What cell types and noncellular features are present in the smear?
ii. What is the most likely diagnosis in the cat?
iii. What ancillary tests should be used to confirm the diagnosis?
iv. What predisposing factors should be considered?

25 i. The main differential diagnoses are naso-pharyngeal polyps, foreign bodies, neoplasia, and infections. However, neoplasia occurs primarily in old cats, with the exception of lymphoma, which may occur in young, especially FeLV positive, cats. Polyps, foreign bodies, and bacterial and fungal infections all commonly cause nasal discharge. Bacteria and fungi may also produce nasal swelling across the bridge of the nose.

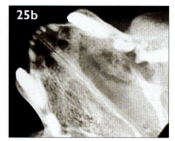

ii. A thorough oral examination, complete blood count, biochemistry panel, urinalysis, and FeLV and FIV tests should all be done. Imaging of the skull is useful to detect bony lysis and increased density in the nasal cavity (**25b**). Cross-sectional imaging such as CT or MRI, if available, is more sensitive, but conventional radiography may be sufficient. After the site and extent of the lesion are identified, a fine-needle aspirate should be performed for culture and cytology. When lesions originate in the caudal portion of the nasal cavity, clinical signs may be subtle. In this case, intraoral radiographs showed a fluid-filled opacity in the left nasal cavity, without nasal septum destruction.

26 i. The sample from the lesion contains many neutrophils, few erythrocytes, numerous epithelial cells, and numerous encapsulated yeast organisms consistent with *Cryptococcus* spp.

ii. Cryptococcosis is caused by *Cryptococcus* spp., ubiquitous yeasts commonly isolated from soil, dust, insects, feces of pigeons, and other avian droppings. In cats, *Cryptococcus neoformans* is more common than *C. gattii*, and the most frequently observed problems are rhinitis or sinusitis with unilateral or bilateral nasal discharge, CNS manifestations, and cutaneous lesions. Nasal discharge is not always present. Other clinical findings may include lymphadenopathy, cough and occasionally dyspnea, chorioretinitis, and other ocular lesions.

iii. Cytologic examination is a quick method to demonstrate the agent from tissue aspirates, impression smears, CSF, and aqueous humor. The agent cannot be visualized in approximately 25% of cases; thus, a negative result in the cytologic examination does not rule out the diagnosis of cryptococcosis. The serum cryptococcal antigen test detects antigens associated with the fungal capsule and is sensitive and specific. Diagnosis can also by confirmed by histopathologic examination of tissue biopsies or culture of the organism.

iv. The predisposing factors for feline cryptococcosis are uncertain. Although FeLV and FIV infections can cause immunosuppression, they are not specifically associated with cryptococcosis. Some reports, however, suggest that cats infected with FeLV or FIV have a higher likelihood of treatment failure than uninfected cats.

27 A 2-year-old castrated male domestic longhair cat was seen because of lethargy of 1 week duration. The cat originally came from Sweden. The owner had moved to Germany 2 months ago and had brought the cat with her from Sweden. On the blood smear, structures were found in the red blood cells (27).

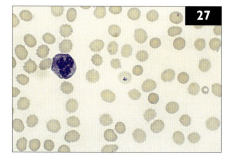

i. What are the structures seen in the red blood cells?

ii. What are the clinical signs of this disease in cats?

iii. What is the treatment for this disease in cats?

28 A 1-year-old spayed female Siamese cat was seen because of sneezing, nasal discharge, bilateral blepharospasm, and ocular discharge. The cat lived indoors and outdoors in a multiple-cat household, and had a complete vaccination history. On physical examination, the only abnormal finding was that the right eye was very red and swollen. Ophthalmic examination revealed that a serous-mucoid ocular discharge, conjunctival hyperemia, and severe chemosis were present in both eyes (28a), with the right eye being more severely affected (28b). The slit lamp examination and the fundic examination were normal in both eyes. Schirmer tear test results were >25 mm/min for the right eye and 16 mm/min for the left eye. Fluorescein staining was negative in both eyes.

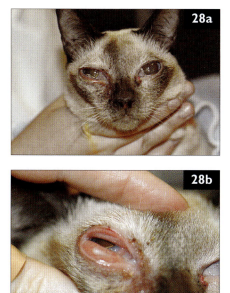

i. What was the problem in this cat?

ii. What was the most likely cause of the problem?

27 i. The parasites in the red blood cells are *Babesia* spp. In domestic cats, *Babesia felis* (South Africa, Sudan), *Babesia cati* (India), and *Babesia canis* subspecies *presentii* (Israel) have been described. Also, *Babesia* spp. have been identified in wild *Felidae* in Africa, including *Babesia herpailuri*, *Babesia leo*, and *Babesia pantherae*. Vectors of *Babesia* spp. in cats are unknown. No cases from Northern Europe have been reported, and it remained unclear how this cat was infected in Sweden or Germany.

ii. Reports of clinical signs in cats with babesiosis come predominantly from South Africa. Usually, cats with naturally occurring babesiosis are younger than 3 years. Clinical signs include lethargy, anorexia, weakness, rough hair coat, diarrhea, anemia, and icterus. Icterus is mainly prehepatic and caused by hemolysis. Anemia can be severe and is probably the reason for lethargy, anorexia, weakness, and the rough hair coat. The disease is usually chronic in cats, and signs may not be apparent for weeks to months.

iii. Treatment of feline babesiosis is not clearly established. Most babesiacidal drugs are ineffective. Primaquine phosphate, an antimalarial compound, seems to be effective and is the drug of choice. However, the effective dose, 0.5 mg/kg PO or intramuscularly (IM), is very close to the lethal dose of 1 mg/kg, so it has to be administered carefully, and only after a definite diagnosis has been made.

28 i. The cat had conjunctivitis, which is a very common problem in cats.

ii. The most important etiologic agents include FHV, *Chlamydophila felis*, and *Mycoplasma* spp. The clinical signs caused by those organisms are usually very similar: blepharospasm, conjunctival hyperemia, chemosis, prolapse of the third eyelid, pain, and ocular discharge, but the following may be useful in their differentiation: FHV is very common; animals in multiple-cat households and catteries have an increased risk for infection. In severe cases of herpes conjunctivitis, the risk of symblepharon formation is very high, especially in young cats. Once infected, cats become latent carriers of the virus and recurrent episodes of conjunctivitis and keratitis may be observed. Cats up to 1 year of age have a significantly higher risk of infection with *Chlamydophila felis* than do older cats. Unilateral conjunctivitis is usually seen, with the second eye being involved a few days later. Conjunctival hyperemia, severe chemosis, and serous to mucopurulent discharge are the most common ocular findings. Younger cats housed in large groups are particularly sensitive to infection with *Mycoplasma* spp. Very often, infection with FHV or other stressors increase the risk of infection. Conjunctivitis may initially be unilateral, but the second eye may also become affected later. Mycoplasmal conjunctivitis is characterized by chemosis, thick mucoid, sticky discharge, and the formation of pseudomembranes on the conjunctival surface.

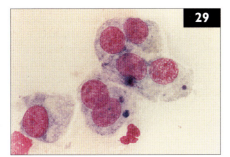

29 Case 29 is the same cat as case 28. A conjunctival scraping and cytology were performed on the right eye (29).
i. Based on cytology, what is the etiologic diagnosis?
ii. What is the treatment of choice for this cat?

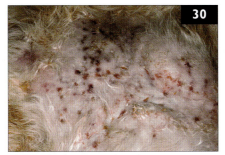

30 A 5-year-old spayed female domestic shorthair cat was seen because of nodular dermatitis that was first noticed 12 months ago. Initially, small nonpruritic nodules had been present. With time they increased in size, and some ulcerated and discharged purulent material. 3 months ago, the cat was treated with antibiotics, with no response. The cat was current on vaccinations and regularly wormed. It had free access to outdoors. There were no other pets in the household. Physical examination showed no other abnormalities. Papules, nodules, and plaques were palpable in the skin of the inguinal area and the inner thighs; a number of them showed draining tracts, and a purulent discharge (without any evidence of granules) could be obtained by applying pressure to the lesions (30).
i. What are the cat's main differential diagnoses?
ii. What are the first tests that should be done?
iii. What is an appropriate further diagnostic plan?

29 i. Within the conjunctival epithelial cells on this slide are multiple intracytoplasmic and basophilic (purple) staining inclusion bodies, typical of an infection with *Chlamydophila felis*. The elementary bodies (infectious form) within the cell can be observed for up to 50 days, but are especially frequent in the first 2 weeks post-infection. Conjunctival cytology is a very easy and helpful diagnostic technique and should be routinely performed in cats with conjunctivitis. A microbrush is swiped across the inferior cul-de-sac and then gently smeared on a glass slide. The slides are dried and fixed in acetone, and then stained with a Romanowsky-type or Giemsa stain.

ii. Treatment of choice for conjunctivitis caused by *C. felis* is topical tetracycline applied to both eyes three to four times daily until resolution of clinical symptoms, and then for an additional week. Alternatively oral doxcyline (10 mg/kg q 24 h) for 3–4 weeks may be administered, which has been shown to clear the infection. This also puts the likely systemic nature of *C. felis* infection into consideration. Enrofloxacin is as effective as doxycycline against *C. felis* but can be associated with retinal toxicity (e.g. in higher dosages) and should only be used if no alternative options are available.

30 i. With any nodular disease in cats the three major groups of disorders to consider are: (1) infectious diseases, (2) sterile inflammation, and (3) neoplastic disease. In the first group, organisms such as *Staphylococcus intermedius*, *Curvularia geniculata*, *Pseudoallescheria boydii*, and, occasionally, *Nocardia* spp. and *Actinomyces* spp., may be found. Also, atypical mycobacteria such as *Mycobacterium fortuitum* or *M. smegmatis* may be seen. Sterile panniculitis and sterile pyogranulomatous dermatitis may be seen and can only be diagnosed by negative culture, failure to respond to trial therapy with antibiotics, and compatible histopathologic changes. This cat is fairly young for neoplastic disease, and neither the site nor the presence of draining tracts are typical of common feline cutaneous neoplasms.

ii. Cytologic evaluation of the purulent discharge is the first step. If neutrophils, macrophages, and organisms are found, an infectious etiology is likely. A finding of pyogranulomatous inflammation without evidence of organisms suggests the need for special stains (acid-fast and fungal stains). Also, bacterial and fungal cultures should be submitted. If neoplastic disease is suspected, histopathologic evaluation of skin biopsies should be performed.

iii. A skin biopsy is the next diagnostic step, and multiple specimens from a variety of lesion must be obtained. Biopsy punches are not the best tool as they fail to provide deep material; excisional biopsies down to the panniculus are better.

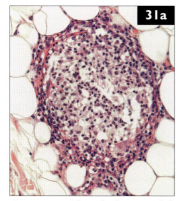

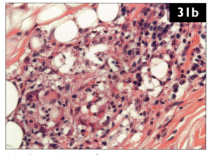

31 Case 31 is the same cat as case 30. Biopsy revealed a pyogranulomatous dermatitis and panniculitis. Bacterial organisms were identified on acid-fast stains in low (31a) and high magnification (31b), and the bacterial culture revealed *Mycobacterium fortuitum* sensitive to doxycycline, enrofloxacin, and a few other antibiotics.
i. What is the prognosis for this cat?
ii. What are the treatment options in this patient?
iii. Which of these options has the highest chance of cure?

32 A 14-month-old intact female Siamese cat was seen because of a 3-week history of diarrhea. It had been acquired from an animal shelter, and had been vaccinated against FPV, FHV, and FCV. It was kept completely indoors. There was a history of an elevated body temperature (39.9°C) once prior to presentation. Physical examination was normal with the exception of bilateral pelvic limb ataxia. Therefore, a complete neurologic examination was performed, which showed decreased proprioceptive positioning, hopping, and extensor postural thrust in both pelvic limbs. Patellar and flexor reflexes were normal. The anus appeared dilated, and there was no anal reflex. CSF was obtained *via* cisternal puncture

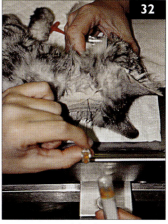

under general anesthesia (32). Analysis revealed an increased leukocyte count (340 cells/µl) and increased CSF protein (1.8 g/l).
i. What are the problems?
ii. What are possible differential diagnoses?
iii. What further test is indicated?

31 i. The prognosis for atypical mycobacterial infections is often considered to be poor, as organisms are not easily eliminated by antimicrobial therapy. Surgical excision of affected tissue frequently leads to wound dehiscence and relapse. However, with prolonged antimicrobial therapy, the prognosis is fair.
ii. One option is antimicrobial therapy. Rifampin, fluoroquinolones, macrolides, tetracyclines, and clofazimine are commonly used drugs; a combination of antibiotics is best. Clinical improvement should be expected within the first 4 weeks; typically, the first change is a decrease in drainage. If there is a positive clinical response to antibiotics, therapy should be continued long-term (6–12 months) and for at least 1–2 months after clinical cure. Unfortunately, bacterial survival in the center of the scar tissue may lead to recurrence.

Alternatively, surgery may be employed. Wide margins are essential, as bacteria may be found beyond the outer edges of the lesion, and flaps or grafts are often required. Such surgery should only be attempted by experienced surgeons. Recurrence of draining tracts is common if adjuvant antibiotic therapy is not used.
iii. The best approach is a combination of the two. Typically, antimicrobial therapy is administered for 4–8 weeks before surgery. The affected tissue is then aggressively excised so that most of the remaining organisms are eliminated. Antimicrobial therapy is continued for at least 2–4 months after wound healing.

32 i. There are three major problems: (1) Diarrhea. (2) Neurologic disease of the pelvic limbs and anus. The neurologic examination suggests there are multifocal lesions involving the T3–L3 and S1–S3 spinal cord segments or nerve roots. (3) There is a history of an elevated body temperature once.
ii. Possible differentials include: (1) Diarrhea in young cats can have a multitude of causes. Here, reduced anal reflex indicates neurolgic disease. Alternatively, multisystemic disease like FIP, lymphoma, or toxoplasmosis could be affecting the spinal cord/cauda equina and the gastrointestinal tract simultaneously. (2) Multifocal spinal cord disease in a young cat could be due to myelitis or meningomyelitis, discospondylitis, intervertebral disk disease, trauma, malformation or hereditary neurodegenerative disease. (3) Elevated body temperature could be either hyperthermia or fever.
iii. The CSF had a marked pleocytosis which was accompanied by increased CSF protein. Thus, the cat was suffering from meningomyelitis. Further information about possible underlying causes of CNS inflammation is commonly obtained from cytologic evaluation of CSF. In the present case, there was a mixed cell population with about 80% neutrophils with a few macrophages, monocytes, and lymphocytes. A mixed cell pattern with high leukocyte count and protein is most indicative of FIP. Rare differentials would be chronic bacterial meningomyelitis or malacia. In this cat, neurologic signs progressed despite antibiotic therapy; FIP was confirmed postmortem.

33 A 7-year-old castrated male domestic shorthair cat was seen because of pelvic limb paresis (33). This had started 6 months ago and progressed considerably. The cat had repeatedly tested positive for FeLV antigen previously. The physical examination was unremarkable apart from the neurologic signs. The hind limbs were extended

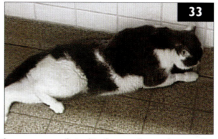

when the cat was in lateral recumbency. There was pelvic limb ataxia and paresis. Intermittently, both pelvic limbs would be dragged behind the body. There was decreased proprioception, hopping, and extensor postural thrust of both pelvic limbs. Proprioceptive positioning and initiation of hopping were also slightly delayed in the right thoracic limb. There was mild anisocoria, with the left pupil larger than the right. The menace response was normal, but direct and consensual pupillary light reflexes were diminished in both eyes.
i. What is the neuroanatomical localization of the disease process in this patient?
ii. What are possible differential diagnoses?

34 Case 34 is the same cat as case 33. It tested positive for FeLV antigen again (34).
i. What diagnostic procedures should be performed?
ii. What is the most likely diagnosis if all diagnostic procedures are unhelpful?

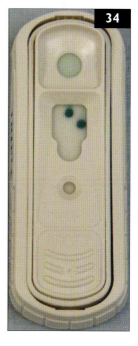

33 i. Abnormal gait in the pelvic limbs with normal pelvic limb spinal reflexes suggests a T3–L3 spinal cord lesion. Additional subtle postural deficits in the right thoracic limb suggest a right-sided cervical spinal cord or brainstem lesion, or a left forebrain lesion. Diminished pupillary light reflexes with normal vision suggests additional involvement of the midbrain, oculomotor nerve, ciliary ganglia, or postganglionic ciliary nerves. Thus, a multifocal or diffuse lesion in the central nervous system (CNS) involving the thoracolumbar spinal cord and midbrain appears most likely. The cat may also have two separate conditions: T3–L3 disease accounting for the pelvic limb paresis, and a second intracranial disease. However, multifocal disease would explain all the neurologic deficits.

ii. Chronic progressive multifocal spinal cord and brainstem disease can be caused by chronic inflammatory disease (e.g. FIP, polioencephalomyelitis, toxoplasmosis, Borna disease, spongiform encephalopathy), multifocal neoplasia, or degenerative conditions. Storage diseases, or other hereditary disorders, anatomic anomalies, and FIP are less likely in cats of this age. Degenerative myelopathy with chronic progressive pelvic limb paresis, ataxia, and abnormal pupillary light reflexes has been described in cats persistently infected with FeLV. Spinal lymphoma and secondary immunosuppressive infection may also be considered in FeLV-infected cats.

34 i. (1) Complete blood count, biochemical profile, and urinalysis should be performed to screen for evidence of inflammation, atypical lymphocytes, or cytopenias due to bone marrow involvement. (2) Spinal radiographs are indicated to screen for disk disease, previous fractures, or neoplasms involving the vertebrae and causing compressive spinal cord disease. (3) Abdominal ultrasound can show evidence of extraneural lymphoma. (4) MRI of the brain and spinal cord may show evidence of thoracolumbar spinal cord compression associated with disk protrusions or neoplasia. This is preferable to myelography because it may also detect intramedullary neoplasms and syringomyelia. (5) Cerebrospinal fluid (CSF) analysis is routinely performed following MRI to diagnose CNS inflammation.

ii. Degenerative myelopathy. This has been reported to occur in cats, usually more than 4 years old, that are persistently infected with FeLV. The clinical signs consist predominately of ataxia, hyperesthesia, and paresis, progressing to paralysis. Some cats also show weakness, lethargy, abnormal behavior, anisocoria with a diminished pupillary light reflex, and urinary incontinence. This disease has a chronic progressive course. In the present case, degenerative myelopathy was suspected because of chronic FeLV p27 antigenemia in the presence of a chronic progressive disease with multifocal neurologic signs. Further support was given by negative results on laboratory, MRI, and CSF examination. Neither immunosuppressive nor immunomodulating therapy appeared to influence the disease course, and the cat was euthanized.

35 A 1-year-old castrated male domestic shorthair cat was seen because of alopecia, crusting, and focal ulceration in the preauricular area due to self trauma (35). The cat had been obtained from a shelter 2 months earlier, at which time it had been vaccinated and wormed. The cat now lived strictly indoors, and was fed dry cat food. It began to scratch its ears severely soon after moving. The other cat in the

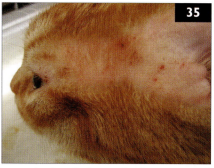

household, an 8-year-old spayed female domestic shorthair cat, had no reported problems. Physical examination showed no abnormalities other than bilateral skin lesions in the preauricular areas and the cheeks. Bilateral otitis externa was also present, characterized by brownish debris in the ear canals.
i. What are the most likely causes of otitis externa in this cat?
ii. What is the best diagnostic approach?

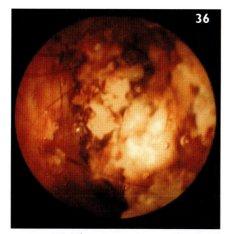

36 Case 36 is the same cat as 35. The otoscopic examination is difficult and neither tympanum can be visualized due to the huge amounts of debris (36). All diagnostic tests are normal or negative.
i. What is the most likely diagnosis if all tests are negative?
ii. What are the treatment options if all tests are negative?

35 i. Preauricular pruritus is frequently associated with otitis externa, which is most frequently caused by ectoparasites or allergies. *Notoedres cati* and *Otodectes cynotis* are the most likely ectoparasites. As these lesions are bilateral and occurred while the cat was living indoors, foreign bodies are less likely, although cat litter granules may cause chronic otitis externa.

ii. Firstly, a smear of the debris in the ear canal should be examined for the presence of *N. cati* or *O. cynotis*. Secondly, another slide from the ear canal debris should be stained and examined for signs of inflammation, and the presence of bacteria or yeasts. Thirdly, impression smears should be obtained from ulcerated skin foci and examined for bacteria and yeasts. However, bacterial infections are typically secondary to another disease and thus, a search for the underlying cause is indicated. Finally, a skin scraping of the affected preauricular skin should be performed, to look for mites. Superficial skin scrapings are performed by applying paraffin oil to the skin and gently scraping it off onto a slide. Deep skin scrapings for *Demodex* spp. mites (although an uncommon cause of aural pruritus in the cat) are taken after the superficial scrape has been performed, by squeezing the skin prior to sampling and then scraping until capillary bleeding is seen.

36 i. The clinical presence of otitis externa with excessive debris in the external canal supports a diagnosis of *Otodectes cynotis* infestation, even if debris analysis and skin scrapings are negative. The cat may have been infected in the shelter and only developed clinical signs later or may have been infected by the other cat in the household, in which case it would be an asymptomatic carrier.

ii. Both cats should be treated with ectoparasiticidal drugs. Topical selemectin and moxidectin are safe and user-friendly treatment options registered in many countries for the treatment of superficial ectoparasites. Topical therapy with systemic activity is preferred in suspected or diagnosed *O. cynotis* infestations as these mites are not necessarily confined to the ear canal and local therapy may miss those mites and/or eggs which are currently residing elsewhere on the body. Alternatively, topical fipronil could be used; with this treatment, one drop should be applied in each ear and the rest of the tube between the shoulder blades to optimize treatment results. In addition to this treatment, an ear flush under anesthesia may be suggested to remove the debris and evaluate the tympanic membranes. That would also allow cytologic sampling of the horizontal canal, which may harbor an infection even if the vertical canal is normal.

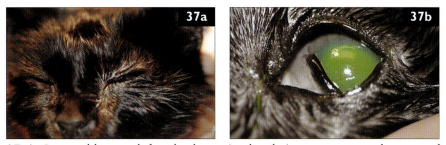

37 A 5-year-old spayed female domestic shorthair cat was seen because of blepharospasm and excessive tearing in the left eye for several days (**37a**). The cat had had a dental operation approximately 1 week before the onset of ocular symptoms. It lived in a multiple-cat household, had outdoor access, and was current on all vaccinations. There had been no previous ocular problems, but the cat had had a severe upper respiratory tract infection as a kitten. Ocular examination revealed the following in the left eye: blepharospasm and tearing; all ocular reflexes were normal; the Schirmer tear test result was >25 mm/min; and the IOP was 10 mmHg. The anterior chamber, lens, and fundus were normal. The eye was stained with fluorescein (**37b**).
i. What is the appearance with fluorescein?
ii. What is the most likely etiology?
iii. What tests could be performed to confirm the diagnosis?
iv. What is the treatment?

38 Two 12-week-old female domestic shorthair kittens were seen because of a history of generalized ataxia, stumbling, and falling since the cats started walking. The cats were from a litter of six with three kittens affected. Both kittens had a broad-based stance, symmetric hypermetria of all four limbs (**38**), and generalized ataxia, none of which had

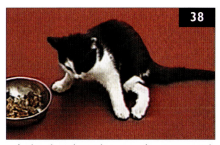

worsened. There was a coarse tremor of the head and truncal sway, with intermittent falling to either side. The head tremor was most pronounced when the cats were offered food. Neurologic examination was otherwise normal except for absent menace responses in both eyes.
i. What is the neuroanatomical localization of the neurologic signs?
ii. What are the differential diagnoses?
iii. What is the pathogenesis of cerebellar hypoplasia in cats?

37 i. Fluorescein staining reveals a large superficial corneal ulcer in the left eye. The cornea is mildly edematous with very fine vessels approaching from the dorsal limbus.

ii. Infection with FHV-1 is most likely. This is the most important corneal pathogen in cats. In adults, FHV infection is frequently caused by reactivation of latent virus, which can be triggered by several stress factors, including anesthesia. Primary infection usually occurs at a young age and may manifest as upper respiratory tract infection. The virus persists lifelong within neural ganglia.

iii. Diagnostic tests for FHV include virus isolation, PCR, or immunofluorescence; PCR is probably the most reliable test here. There may also be infection with FeLV or FIV, and testing for those viruses is indicated if the status is unknown. Corneal or conjunctival cytology may also be helpful to identify any concurrent ocular diseases.

iv. Topical antiviral drugs should be used. Idoxuridine, trifluridine, and vidarabine are the most effective in cats. Topical antibiotics should also be used to prevent secondary bacterial infection. Ocular inflammation and pain can be successfully treated with nonsteroidal anti-inflammatory drugs. Topical corticosteroids are absolutely contraindicated. Also, corneal ulcers with loose epithelial edges should be carefully debrided with a dry cotton tip to encourage healing.

38 i. The neurologic examination findings indicate cerebellar disease. This is characterized by normal mental status and symmetric ataxia with hypermetric movements of the limbs, trunk, and head. 'Intention tremor' is often a feature: tremor which typically is exaggerated by goal-oriented movements. Absent menace responses may also be a feature, but these may be normal in kittens up to 12 weeks of age.

ii. Cerebellar disease in more than one kitten from the same litter suggests a congenital disorder. Two types of congenital cerebellar disease are possible; they can be distinguished by the course of the disease: (1) Nonprogressive cerebellar ataxia; this is caused by malformations such as cerebellar hypoplasia and is first evident when the kittens start to walk. The ataxia persists throughout life. (2) Chronic progressive cerebellar ataxia. Causes include inherited neurodegenerative disorders like cerebellar abiotrophy, neuroaxonal dystrophy, or storage disorders (GM1 and GM2 gangliosidosis, sphingomyelinosis, and mannosidosis). Neurologic signs are first seen in kittens or young adult cats less than 12 months of age and gradually progress. Inflammatory CNS disease, often caused by the FIP virus, can also cause progressive cerebellar disease and should be excluded in cats with progressive cerebellar signs. In the present case, the history and clinical signs pointed towards cerebellar hypoplasia as the most likely cause.

iii. In kittens, this is most commonly caused by *in utero* exposure to FPV. Often, only some kittens in a litter are affected.

39 A 3-year-old spayed female domestic shorthair cat was seen because of signs of purulent nasal discharge that had been present since the owner adopted the cat from an animal shelter 2 weeks earlier. This had not improved with a 10-day course of amoxicillin/clavulanate. The vaccination status was unknown. The owner reported the cat had a decreased appetite and activity level,

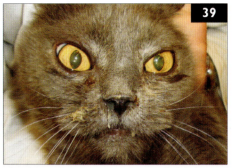

and open-mouth breathing when stressed. Physical examination revealed bilateral purulent nasal discharge (39), marked inspiratory nasal stridor, and inspiratory dyspnea when the patient was manipulated. Otherwise, the physical examination was normal. A CT scan of the nose revealed almost total loss of intranasal turbinates and thickening of the nasal mucosa. Retrograde rhinoscopic imaging of the nasopharynx demonstrated white irregularly-shaped masses adherent to the mucosal surface. Biopsy samples were obtained for histopathology and microbiological testing.

i. What is the most likely diagnosis in this patient?
ii. Which diagnostic tests are helpful?

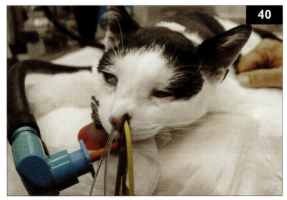

40 Case 40 is the same cat as case 39. Aspergillosis was diagnosed in this cat.
i. Discuss treatment options including the procedure shown (40).
ii. What are potential risk factors associated with these treatment modalities?

39 i. Aspergillosis is most likely – infection with the fungus *Aspergillus* spp., which is rare in cats. Aspergillosis is considered an opportunistic infection, since *Aspergillus* spp. are present in the mucous membranes of healthy animals. The lack of clinical response to antibiotic treatment suggests a fungal cause. The CT and rhinoscopic findings are also highly suggestive of aspergillosis.

ii. Confirmation of this often requires multiple tests. Because *Aspergillus* spp. can be found in the normal nasal cavity, a positive fungal culture from a nasal swab is not sufficient to diagnose the disease. Clinical signs and results obtained from CT and rhinoscopy can be suspicious, but further tests are indicated to establish a definite diagnosis. No information is available about the diagnostic usefulness of *Aspergillus* spp. antibody tests in cats, although these can be helpful in dogs with nasal aspergillosis. Here, antibody tests are often negative at the start of the disease, but they can aid in establishing a diagnosis when positive. To confirm the diagnosis, biopsy specimens from abnormal nasal tissue, ideally obtained endoscopically under direct visualization, should be submitted for histopathology, imprint cytology, and fungal culture. If one of these diagnostic methods is positive for *Aspergillus* spp, in combination with the presence of typical clinical signs and characteristic findings on endoscopy and CT, sinonasal aspergillosis is very likely.

40 i. Not much information is available about treatment modalities for nasal aspergillosis in cats. A combination of local and systemic therapy is recommended. Before local intranasal therapy is started, intranasal fungal plaques should be removed endoscopically or surgically. Then, clotrimazole (1% in propylene glycol) should be infused intranasally. This has been performed extensively in dogs, but has only been utilized in a few cats. The cat is anesthetized and intubated, and foley catheters are placed to occlude the nasopharynx and nares (**40**). The nasopharynx and paranasal sinuses are then slowly infused by syringe for an hour. The pharynx should be packed with gauze sponges to prevent aspiration of the infusate, which must be fully removed from the pharynx and larynx at the end of the procedure, before the tube is removed. In addition to intranasal infusion, systemic antifungal therapy should be administered for at least 4 months; itraconazole is the drug of choice. The starting dose (10 mg/kg q 24 h) should be reduced if side-effects occur.

ii. Potential side-effects of itraconazole treatment can be hepatotoxicity, increased ALT activity, weight loss, and anorexia. If side-effects occur, the dose should be reduced. Intranasal instillation of clotrimazole can lead to slight irritation and nasal discharge for several days after the procedure. Cases of pulmonary edema have also been reported in cats following the procedure; these might have been caused by leakage and aspiration of clotrimazole.

41 A 6-year-old castrated male domestic shorthair cat was seen because of a history of chronic vomiting of 6 months' duration. The cat lived indoors only. Physical examination, hematology, biochemistry, abdominal radiographs and ultrasound examination were unremarkable. Endoscopic biopsies were obtained from the gastric mucosa (**41**).

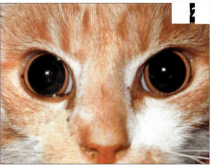

i. Which organism can be identified?
ii. How else can this organism be diagnosed in cats?
iii. Which species of this organism are most commonly seen in cats?
iv. Is this organism a pathogen?

42 A 3-year-old spayed female domestic shorthair cat was referred for a suspected upper respiratory tract infection. It had been initially seen for bilateral nasal discharge and had been treated with amoxicillin/clavulanate (20 mg/kg PO q 12 h), but this failed to produce a favorable clinical response. The cat subsequently was treated with corticosteroids, but deteriorated markedly. It developed bilaterally dilated pupils,

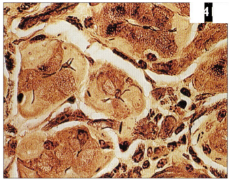

which failed to respond to bright light (**42**), blindness, signs of vestibular disease (e.g. loss of balance, falling, positional nystagmus), and seizures.
i. What neuroanatomical lesions can result in blindness associated with bilaterally dilated pupils that fail to respond to light?
ii. What diagnostic tests can help differentiate the possible causes of this type of blindness?
iii. What inferences can be drawn from concurrent vestibular signs, seizures, and bilaterally dilated pupils, with respect to the cat's underlying neurologic disease?
iv. What are the cat's two main problems, and can both problems be explained by a common etiology?
v. What are the differential diagnoses?

41 i. This is a Warthin–Starry-stained slide demonstrating *Helicobacter* spp. organisms in the gastric glands.
ii. At present, diagnosis of *Helicobacter* spp. in veterinary patients requires invasive testing (i.e. gastric biopsy). In addition to histopathology, *Helicobacter* spp. are most commonly diagnosed by rapid urease testing of gastric mucosal biopsy specimens. Although not commonly available, PCR testing of gastric biopsies and fecal samples from cats (and dogs) has been reported experimentally. Only culture and PCR testing allow identification of the particular *Helicobacter* species present. Also, a positive clinical response to antibiotic therapy supports the belief that bacteria are a cause of the clinical signs.
iii. *H. felis, H. heilmannii, H. bizzozeronii, H. pametensis*, and *H. pylori* have all been reported in cats; infections with multiple species are possible.
iv. At the moment, it is unknown whether all veterinary *Helicobacter* species are pathogens, and whether there is a difference in virulence between different pathogenic species. Therefore, the role of *Helicobacter* spp. in the development of gastrointestinal disease in cats is unknown; further research is needed.

42 i. Blindness associated with bilaterally dilated pupils that fail to respond to light is, by definition, peripheral blindness, and therefore, the result of disease of the retinas, optic nerves, optic chiasm, or optic tracts.
ii. The best way to sort out these various possibilities is by direct or indirect ophthalmoscopy (preferably the latter). In this cat, there was retinitis, with hemorrhage around the optic disc resulting in focal retinal detachments. Increased prominence of the optic disc suggested that optic neuritis was present also. In cases in which the retina and optic disc are unremarkable, electroretinography and CT or MRI can be useful.
iii. Vestibular signs indicate disease of the peripheral or central vestibular area; however, positional nystagmus is strongly suggestive of disease of the central vestibular area, i.e. the brainstem in the caudal fossa (under the cerebellum). Seizures usually signify disease of telencephalic structures, typically the cerebral cortex. These findings indicate that the cat most likely had multifocal intracranial and intraocular disease.
iv. The cat had two main problems: (1) multifocal intracranial and intraocular disease, and (2) upper respiratory tract disease. In this cat, it is possible that the disease was initially restricted to the nasal cavity and then spread to involve the eyes and CNS following administration of corticosteroids.
v. Fungal and neoplastic diseases are both capable of behaving in this way, but in a young adult cat, cryptococcosis, pheohyphomycosis, *Neosartorya* infection, and lymphoma would be the most likely differential diagnoses. Infections involving *Neosartorya* spp. tend to cause signs of retrobulbar mass unilaterally or bilaterally.

43 Case **43** is the same cat as case **42**. An MRI scan was performed (**43**).
i. What additional diagnostic tests are indicated?
ii. Were the collection of CSF and a scan of the cat's brain using cross-sectional imaging indicated?
iii. Apart from cost, are there any negative aspects to performing these procedures?

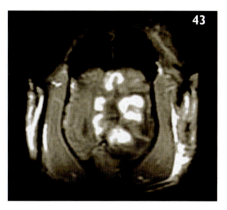

44 Case **44** is the same cat as cases **42** and **43**. *Cryptococcus gattii* was cultured on Sabouraud's glucose agar, and the cat was diagnosed with multiple cerebral cryptococcomas (**44**; fixed brain of another cat which died of cryptococcosis).
i. What is the prognosis in this cat?
ii. How should this cat be treated?

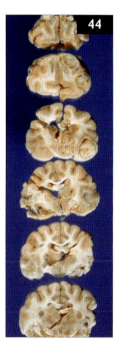

43 i. The simplest, cheapest, and most efficient way to investigate this cat further is to obtain material from the nasal cavity for cytology or histopathology. This is easily performed by obtaining nasal swabs or nasal washings. In this case, cytology from nasal swabs demonstrated large numbers of capsulated, budding yeasts, and *Cryptococcus gattii* was subsequently cultured on Sabouraud's glucose agar. The diagnosis is, therefore, cryptococcal rhinitis with dissemination to the retinas, optic nerves, and CNS.

ii. Not only are nasal swabs or washing a cheaper and easier way to establish a diagnosis in cases such as this, but this approach avoids the need for general anesthesia and CSF collection from a patient with possible increased intracranial pressure. The induction of general anesthesia, and especially CSF collection, often results in marked neurologic deterioration in these patients, so making the diagnosis *via* the nasal cavity has significant advantages. MRI provides useful information concerning whether CNS disease is predominantly meningeal or involves crypto-coccal granulomas (cryptococcomas) in the substance of the brain. MRI was performed in this cat and showed multiple cerebral cryptococcomas.

iii. Although CSF collection and CT or MRI scanning provides useful information, the risk of anesthesia may outweigh the benefits of this additional information in many situations.

44 i. The prognosis is guarded. Cryptococcosis is hard to cure, and cases in which the infection has spread to the CNS are particularly challenging.

ii. Five drugs are useful here: amphotericin B, flucytosine, fluconazole, itraconazole, and terbinafine. Many cases improve with fluconazole or itraconazole, although only fluconazole penetrates the normal blood–brain barrier. Combination therapy is much more effective, using amphotericin B and flucytosine followed by fluconazole (to treat residual foci of infection). Amphotericin B is used SC as a dilute infusion, to delay its absorption into the systemic circulation, thereby avoiding high peak blood levels and sparing the kidneys as a result of maintaining renal perfusion. It is, therefore, possible to administer larger and thus more effective quantities using this protocol than have been administered previously. It is important, however, to monitor plasma urea and creatinine concentrations during therapy. At the completion of this, oral antifungal medication (fluconazole or itraconazole, terbinafine with or without flucytosine) is continued for several months continuing until the antigen titers drop to zero. Some cats may require lifelong treatment with fluconazole to prevent recurrence. This cat achieved a full remission, as reflected by a fall in its antigen titer to zero. Vestibular signs and seizures responded completely to treatment, and the cat regained its sight, although some pupillary dilatation persisted.

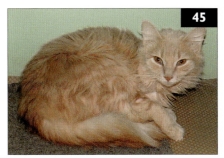

45 A 4-year-old spayed female domestic longhair cat (45) was seen for a consultation. The cat lives in close contact with a 4-year-old neutered male Husky; both cat and dog go outside. The Husky had been diagnosed with leptospirosis caused by the serovar Grippotyphosa and had been in the intensive care unit of the veterinary hospital for the last 2 days. Now, the owner was very concerned about potential infection of the cat.
i. Can cats get leptospirosis?
ii. How are cats usually infected?
iii. Are infected cats a risk for humans or dogs?

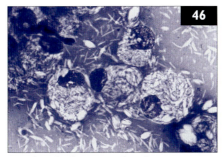

46 A 12-year-old castrated male domestic shorthair cat was seen because of a non-healing wound on its left hock, which had not responded to drainage and 4 weeks' treatment with oral cephalexin then amoxicillin/clavulanate. The cat lived predominantly outdoors, and was known to be FIV-positive. A fine-needle aspirate of the exudate from the wound was obtained and stained with modified Wrights–Giemsa (46).
i. What are the features of the cytology?
ii. What are the differential diagnoses?
iii. How should a definitive diagnosis be obtained?
iv. How should this cat be treated?

45 i. Leptospirosis is caused by infection with antigenically different serovars of the bacterium *Leptospira interrogans*. Although cats can be infected by *Leptospira* spp., clinical illness is very rare. Cats can be exposed to *Leptospira* spp. excreted by wildlife, and *Leptospira* spp. antibodies are present in up to 10% of the feline population. Outdoor cats have a higher likelihood of having antibodies than indoor ones. Serovars *canicola*, *grippotyphosa*, and *pomona* have all been isolated from cats. Although cats develop antibodies after exposure, they appear to be less susceptible than dogs to infections, and clinical signs of feline leptospirosis are usually inapparent or mild.

ii. Unlike dogs, that are usually infected when swimming in *Leptospira*-contaminated water, cats usually become infected through transmission from hunting rodents. They may also be exposed to the urine of cohabitating dogs.

iii. Although cats can be infected experimentally, they do not seem to remain chronic carriers. Thus, an antibody-positive cat does not seem to be a major zoonotic risk when compared with dogs, that may shed organisms for a long time. Furthermore, the majority of leptospiral infections in humans and dogs are contracted while engaging in water-related activities. As most cats dislike water, they pose little risk of causing disease transmission.

46 i. There are large macrophages present, with masses of negatively-staining bacilli in their cytoplasm.

ii. Infection with *Mycobacterium* spp. is most likely. Negative staining of bacteria within macrophages on modified Wright–Giemsa stains is a characteristic of mycobacterial infection. Abundant intracellular bacteria are characteristic of the lepromatous form of feline leprosy, caused by *Mycobacterium lepraemurium* and other species of mycobacteria, e.g. *M. visibile*. Cutaneous tuberculosis (*M. bovis*, or rarely *M. avium* or *M. microti*) and atypical mycobacteriosis are less likely differential diagnoses. Disseminated disease is common in the former. Infection with *Nocardia* spp. is possible, but these usually stain positively and branch.

iii. Culture of the causative organism. Although this can be difficult, mycobacterial culture should always be attempted, since it is not possible to distinguish between species on clinical criteria alone. PCR and direct sequencing (if available) is the most reliable and rapid means of identifying mycobacterial species from clinical cases.

iv. Since antimicrobial resistance may occur with single-agent therapy, the best treatment regime is multi-agent antimicrobial therapy using a combination of clofazimine or rifampicin with clarithromycin and a fluoroquinolone (e.g. ciprofloxacin). Successful treatment may take 3–6 months and surgical debriding or debulking of lesions is usually necessary. Antibiotic treatment should continue for at least 1–2 months after clinical resolution of lesions.

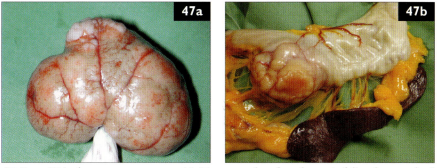

47 Case 47 is the same cat as case 46. Two months after the cat's feline leprosy had been cured, it became anorectic and polydipsic. On physical examination, a cranial abdominal mass was palpated and both kidneys were enlarged, firm, and irregular. The owners declined further investigation and the cat was euthanized. At necropsy, changes in the kidneys (47a), stomach, and spleen (47b) were found.
i. What is the most likely diagnosis?
ii. Could another treatment have been recommended in this case?

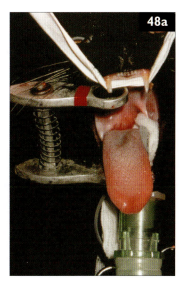

48 A 7-year-old castrated male domestic shorthair cat was seen because of a loss of voice and reluctance to eat over 2–3 weeks, during which time the cat had lost 0.5 kg in body weight. Immediately prior to this, the cat had been 'a bit snuffly'. The owners had noticed that an abnormal respiratory noise was present on inspiration. The cat would lap and swallow liquids, but refused any solid food. On physical examination, the cat had mild inspiratory dyspnea, with flaring of the nostrils and an exaggerated respiratory effort. During examination of the oral cavity, a mass lesion was detected on the right hand side of the nasopharynx, resulting in bulging and ventral displacement of the soft palate (48a).
i. How should the cat be evaluated further, and what would be the most cost-effective way of making a diagnosis?
ii. What treatment is indicated?

47 i. Tumors are shown in the renal cortex and greater curvature of the stomach. Since this cat was FIV-positive, the most likely diagnosis is lymphoma. FIV-positive cats are five to six times as likely to develop lymphoma as uninfected cats. FIV-associated lymphomas are predominantly extranodal, often in unusual sites such as brain, heart, eyes, and spinal cord and often classified as the 'miscellaneous' forms of lymphoma; they are typically high-grade. Usually, FIV has an indirect role in lymphomagenesis, with tumors developing secondary to decreased immune surveillance, polyclonal B cell activation, cytokine production, and/or possibly infectious cofactors. In this case, the omental fat was stained orange from chronic administration of clofazimine for treatment of *M. lepraemurium* infection.

ii. Median remission and survival times for FIV-positive cats with lymphoma are similar to those of FIV-negative cats. In contrast, FeLV infection is a negative prognostic factor in cats with lymphoma. Therefore, multi-agent chemotherapy is indicated in the treatment of lymphoma in FIV-positive cats. However, complications may arise using chemotherapy in cats with FIV infection, especially in those with peripheral cytopenias or concurrent secondary infections. This cat, first seen because of *M. lepraemurium* infection, may have had a late-stage FIV infection then. If chemotherapy had been selected for this cat, it should have also been monitored for recurrence of the mycobacterial infection.

48 i. The cat had a disease of the soft palate, or more likely, the posterior portion of the nasal cavity, and adjacent nasopharynx. The disease appeared to be progressive. The simplest and most cost-effective way of proceeding with this case would be to perform a fine-needle aspirate of the nasopharyngeal mass under general anesthesia. Cytologic evaluation of the smears made from aspirates showed granulomatous inflammation and large numbers of capsulated, budding yeasts in the cat. *Cryptococcus gattii* was subsequently isolated on Sabouraud's agar.

ii. Using diathermy, the soft palate was incised on the midline, and the granuloma dorsal to it was debulked as much as possible (**48b**). The base of the granuloma was curetted, and the wound was closed in two layers using absorbable sutures. The cat was given fluconazole IV intraoperatively, and subsequently treated with itraconazole. The cat immediately improved following surgery, as this operation had relieved the upper airway obstruction and the structural basis for its dysphagia.

Two weeks later, the cat was doing well, but there was still some swelling evident at the site of surgery. The cat continued to do well on this medication, and was treated until the cryptococcal antigen titer had declined to zero. Disease did not recur.

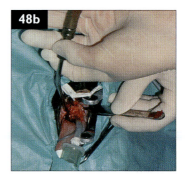

48b

49 A 14-month-old intact male domestic shorthair cat was seen because of a history of multiple skin lumps developing during the past 3 weeks. The cat had been adopted 2 months ago from a group of farm cats. The skin changes had started as nodules, become alopecic, and then ulcerated. The first lesions had been seen on the left antebrachium (49a) and subsequently appeared on the head (49b), neck, toes, ventral abdomen, and prepuce. The physical examination was normal with the exception of the cutaneous lesions, which did not appear to bother the cat.

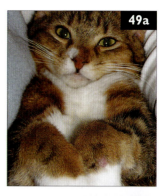

i. What are the differential diagnoses?
ii. How should the diagnosis be obtained?
iii. How is this disease treated?
iv. What is the prognosis?
v. Are there differences in the epidemiology of the different species causing this disease?

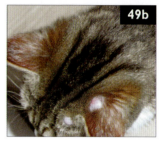

50 A 12-week-old intact female domestic shorthair kitten was seen because of weight loss despite having a normal appetite. The client owned four adult neutered cats, and also fostered cats and kittens from a local shelter, including the kitten that was presented (50), its littermates, and an unrelated cat and her kittens. All of the fostered cats and kittens had contact with each other, but not with the client's own adult cats.

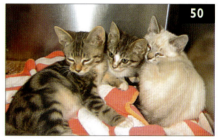

The fostered cats and kittens all tested negative for FeLV antigen and FIV antibody, had been treated for parasites, and had been vaccinated against FPV, FHV, and FCV. The kitten seen was lethargic and had a body temperature of 39.4°C. It developed a distended abdomen, declined further despite antibiotic therapy, and was euthanized. Post-mortem examination showed there was viscous straw-colored fluid in the abdomen.

i. What is the most likely diagnosis?
ii. What relatively cheap test could be done ante-mortem to help make the diagnosis?

49 i. Feline leprosy, cutaneous tuberculosis, atypical mycobacteriosis, actinomycosis, nocardiosis, fungal infections, neoplasia, and eosinophilic granulomas are the main differential diagnoses in this case.

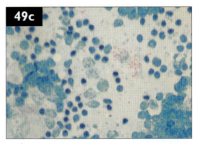

ii. Cytology, histopathology, and culture of the causative organism should be performed. Cytologic analysis of fine-needle aspirates revealed degenerate neutrophils and macrophages. A Ziehl–Neelsen stain identified slender rod-shaped acid-fast organisms located within macrophages and giant cells (49c). Histopathology revealed pyogranulomatous inflammation containing clumps of acid-fast staining organisms. Mycobacterial cultures were negative. However, *Mycobacterium lepraemurium* was diagnosed by PCR, resulting in a presumptive diagnosis of feline leprosy.

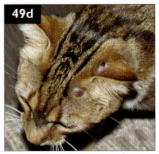

iii. A combination of surgery and drug administration is required. Focal lesions should be removed using a wide surgical excision, and the cat should also be given adjunctive multi-drug antibiotic therapy: clofazamine plus one or both of clarithromycin and rifampicin. Treatment should be continued for 1–2 months after the disappearance of lesions to reduce the risk of recurrence.

iv. *M. lepraemurium* spreads aggressively and often recurs postoperatively if long-term antibiotics are not used. In this cat, lesions on the head became ulcerated (49d) during the course of the disease. All lesions eventually resolved with therapy.

v. Feline leprosy may be caused by *M. haemophilum* or *M. lepraemurium*. The former stains with H&E, but the latter does not. *M. lepraemurium* occurs in younger cats, more often in males, and is contracted *via* the bites of infected rodents; *M. haemophilum* occurs in older and immunosuppressed cats.

50 i. This is a high-density feline 'herd' situation with many kittens that originated from an even more dense shelter situation. The history and physical signs indicate that this kitten most likely succumbed to FIP. Infections with other feline viruses (e.g. FPV, FHV, FCV) should also be considered in a multi-cat situation.

ii. The ascites provided a convenient sample of fluid for testing. A simple and inexpensive test for diagnosing FIP in cats with effusion is the Rivalta test. This test has a positive predictive value of 86% and a negative predictive value of 97%. In shelters, it is often necessary to diagnose based on history, clinical signs, and one or two simple tests, thus, this test should be recommended.

51 Case **51** is the same cat as case 50. The foster parent did not know what to do about the remaining littermates or the fostered queen and her three kittens (**51**). She was also very concerned about her own resident adult cats. Losing foster homes may mean that more kittens will need to be euthanized and widespread panic about FIP can result in decreased feline adoptions from the shelter.

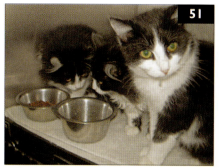

i. What should this foster parent be advised regarding risk of the disease in the littermates?
ii. What should this foster parent be advised regarding risk of the disease in the unrelated foster kittens in the same household?
iii. What should this foster parent be advised regarding risk to the other adult cats in the house?
iv. Can this foster parent safely foster more kittens?

52 A 9-year-old spayed female domestic shorthair cat was seen because of a 4–5-year history of intermittent cough (**52**). Shortly before presentation, it had shown exacerbation of cough and episodes of open-mouth breathing. Previously, it had been managed with prednisolone when the clinical signs worsened. This time, they had not resolved with prednisolone. The cat lived indoors with another indoor cat and was fully vaccinated. On physical examination, the body temperature was 40.2°C; the respiratory rate was 60 bpm, with a prolonged expiratory phase. Heart and respiratory sounds were normal, but when the cat was stressed there was a sudden onset of dyspnea (**BS6**). A complete blood count was performed; the abnormal results were: white blood cells 25.2×10^9/l, mature neutrophils 21.5×10^9/l, band neutrophils 0.8×10^9/l, eosinophils 1.2×10^9/l.

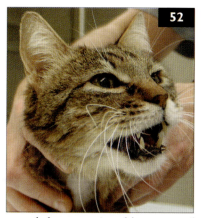

i. What are likely explanations for chronic cough in this cat?
ii. Which further diagnostic testing is recommended?

51 i. Heritability of developing FIP is about 50% so full sibling littermates are twice as likely to develop FIP as other cats. The risk of this occurring depends on genetic factors, age, the strain of FCoV that is circulating, and the immune system and genetics of the individual cat.

ii. The risk for these kittens is lower. Studies have shown that unrelated kittens in households in which FIP has been diagnosed do not have a higher likelihood of developing the disease than kittens in FIP-free households. However, factors that increase FCoV replication and mutation include having multiple cats housed closely together, especially kittens under 1 year of age, and having a more virulent or mutagenic strain of FCoV.

iii. It is likely that all the cats in this household have been exposed to FCoV. The unrelated adult cats are not at higher risk than before of developing FIP due to the reasons mentioned above and, importantly, their age-related resistance.

iv. The foster parent should not foster more kittens after these for at least 3 months. It is always best to foster only one litter at a time to lessen the chance of disease transmission.

52 i. The history, in combination with a positive response to anti-inflammatory treatment, is consistent with a diagnosis of feline asthma. In the present exacerbation of symptoms, eosinophilia could indicate a hypersensitivity reaction. However, the cat also shows fever, and leukocytosis with left shift, indicating bacterial infection. In this case, chronic bronchial disease and immunosuppressive treatment with corticosteroids could have caused structural changes of the airways. If this has occurred, infection can be generated by the normal bacterial microflora of the upper respiratory tract or by primary respiratory bacterial pathogens such as *Bordetella bronchiseptica* or *Mycoplasma* spp.

ii. (1) Thoracic radiographs should be taken. Feline asthma typically shows a predominantly bronchiolar pattern with alveolar involvement in more severe cases, overinflation of the lungs, and sometimes a collapsed right middle lung lobe. (2) A BAL should be performed to gain material for cytology and bacterial culture. BAL cytology is an important diagnostic tool if inflammatory or infectious processes in the lower airways are suspected. Neutrophilic inflammation and intracellular bacteria indicate bacterial infection; eosinophilic inflammation in the absence of bacteria would indicate feline asthma. (3) If radiographs show signs of localized changes within the airways, bronchoscopy is indicated to visualize abnormal areas and obtain sample material from these areas. (4) The cat should also be tested for FeLV and FIV, since these infections can lead to immunosuppression.

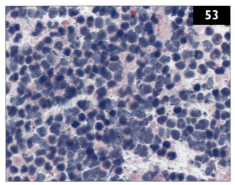

53 Case 53 is the same cat as case 52. Thoracic radiographs of the cat were performed and they showed a bronchial lung pattern. The patient was anesthetized for a BAL performed through a sterile endotracheal tube. Cytologic smears of the sample were prepared (53) and cultures for aerobic bacteria and *Mycoplasma* spp. were performed.

i. What information does cytology provide in this case?

ii. If a bacterial culture of the BAL of this patient is sent to a laboratory and returns negative does this result rule out bacterial infection?

iii. Should antibiotic treatment be started before the results from culture and sensitivity testing are available?

iv. Which antibiotics should be used?

54 Case 54 is the same cat as cases 52 and 53. Three days later, the bacterial culture of the BAL fluid showed heavy growth of *Bordetella bronchiseptica* (54). *Mycoplasma* spp. culture was negative. Antibiotic sensitivity testing indicated that the *B. bronchiseptica* was resistant to all drugs except enrofloxacin and gentamicin.

i. Which of the two antibiotics is preferable in this cat?

ii. Is it recommended to vaccinate the other cat in the household against *B. bronchiseptica*?

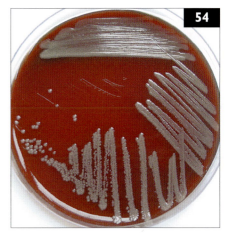

53 i. BAL cytology revealed neutrophilic inflammation with intra- and extracellular rod-shaped bacteria. This fits with a diagnosis of bacterial infection of the lower airways.

ii. Even if the bacterial culture is negative, bacterial infection cannot be ruled out completely. There are multiple causes of a false-negative test result, including: (1) inadequate handling and shipping of the sample, and (2) use of inappropriate culture medium; this is very important if bordetellosis is suspected. Also, since *Mycoplasma* spp. require selective medium for growth, the laboratory should be informed about suspicion of mycoplasmal infection, and samples should be delivered promptly in special transport medium. If cytology of the BAL suggests bacterial infection despite negative bacterial culture, appropriate antibiotic therapy is warranted. If a positive response to antibiotic therapy is observed, this could also indicate bacterial infection.

iii. Antimicrobial treatment should be initiated immediately, because the patient shows severe clinical signs. Empiric antibiotic therapy is indicated to prevent further aggravation of infection. When information is obtained from bacterial culture and sensitivity testing, antibiotic therapy can be modified, if necessary.

iv. Most rod-shaped organisms cultured from the respiratory tract are Gram-negative bacteria, e.g. *Pasteurella* spp., *Escherichia coli*, or *Bordetella bronchiseptica*. Since rod-shaped bacteria were detected on cytology, the chosen antibiotic should have good efficacy against these. Possible choices are fluoroquinolones, aminoglycosides, or third-generation cephalosporins. Also useful in cases of respiratory disease are doxycycline and azithromycin.

54 i. Both drugs can be administered intravenously, which is advantageous in critically ill cats. Enrofloxacin reaches much higher concentrations within the tracheobronchial tree than gentamicin. Fluoroquinolones also have the advantage of accumulation within the neutrophils. However, both drugs can display side-effects. Enrofloxacin may cause acute retinal degeneration in some cats leading to irreversible blindness, and gentamicin can cause nephrotoxicity. Possible alternatives to enrofloxacin are other fluoroquinolones which are less likely to cause retinal damage. If gentamicin is used, renal function should be evaluated before treatment and regularly during treatment. Alternatively, gentamicin could be administered by nebulization, thus reaching a high local concentration within the tracheobronchial tree while reducing the risk of systemic side-effects.

ii. *B. bronchiseptica* is a primary pathogen of the respiratory tract in cats and can cause both upper and lower respiratory tract infections. It is easily transmitted by contact, sneezing, and contaminated equipment. Therefore, infection of the second cat in the household is possible. An intranasal live *B. bronchiseptica* vaccine is available; if used, clinical signs are reduced from 3 days after vaccination. Thus, vaccination of the second cat in the household with an intranasal *B. bronchiseptica* vaccine several days before contact with the infected cat when it returns from the hospital may be beneficial.

55 A 16-month-old neutered female domestic shorthair cat was seen for its annual health check-up in the USA (55). The cat lived primarily indoors, but was allowed to go outside. There were no other cats in the household, but there were several cats in the neighborhood. The cat had received a series of three vaccinations against FPV, FHV, and FCV at 8, 12, and 16 weeks of age; two vaccinations against FeLV at 12 and 16 weeks of age, and one vaccination against rabies at 16 weeks of age. It had negative FeLV and FIV tests at 16 weeks of age. It received selemectin for parasite control, and had been healthy since it was obtained by the owner at 8 weeks of age. Physical examination was unremarkable.

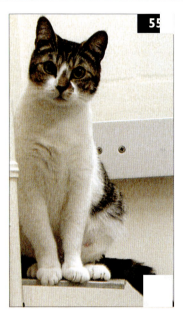

i. Should the cat be vaccinated at this visit?
ii. If so, what vaccines should be administered, and when would booster vaccines be due?

56 A young adult (age unknown) female (sterilization history unknown) domestic shorthair cat in an animal shelter was found severely depressed and dehydrated with green vomit in the cage at the time of morning cleaning (56). It had been in the shelter for 9 days. An adult (age unknown) male (neutering history unknown) domestic shorthair cat housed in the same ward was also vomiting and depressed. It had been in the shelter for 11 days. Both had been

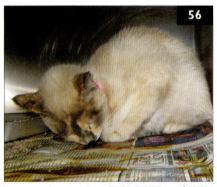

vaccinated on intake with an inactivated virus vaccine against FPV, FHV, and FCV SC. According to cleaning staff, no abnormalities were noticed in either cat the previous afternoon, and both had been described as apparently healthy on intake.
i. What are the most likely differential diagnoses for this condition?
ii. What diagnostic tests could be performed in-house to provide additional information?
iii. How could a definitive diagnosis be made?

55 i. As a kitten, the cat received an appropriate series of core vaccines (FPV, FHV, FCV, rabies) administered over a time period likely to be sufficient to avoid interference from passively acquired maternal antibodies. Core booster vaccines should be administered 1 year following the primary immunization series.

ii. A general principle of vaccination is to provide protection against important pathogens while minimizing the risk of adverse reactions. Thus, the health and lifestyle of each cat should be individually assessed to select a vaccination protocol tailored to its needs using the minimum number of vaccines possible. In this cat, core vaccine boosters (FPV, FHV, FCV) should be administered now to protect against these common and highly infectious diseases. These vaccines induce very durable immunity lasting a minimum of 3 years, and probably longer. Concerning rabies vaccination, the regulations of each individual jurisdiction have to be considered. Since this cat roams outdoors and may have contact with other cats of unknown FeLV infection status, FeLV vaccination is advisable in most countries in which FeLV infection is endemic. The duration of immunity induced by FeLV vaccines is less clear than for the other antigens. A reasonable approach in this cat (living in the USA) would be to vaccinate against FPV, FHV, FCV, FeLV, and rabies at this visit, and recommend a 3-year interval before the next vaccines are administered.

56 i. In a shelter cat, the most likely infectious cause is FPV infection. Also, *Salmonella* spp.-infected cats can present similarly.

ii. A patient-side test for parvovirus antigen can be used to detect FPV in feces. However, this can give false-positive results in recently vaccinated cats. Occasional false-negatives can also occur (e.g. if the feces are very watery), so this should not be ruled out on the basis of a fecal test alone. A blood smear to estimate white blood cell count can also be done in-house. Both FPV infection and salmonellosis can cause depressed white cell counts, so this would not differentiate between them. However, if the white blood cell count appears normal or elevated, other diagnoses may be more likely. If a cat dies or is euthanized, an in-house necropsy should be performed. Segmental enteritis suggests feline parvovirosis, but an absence of gross lesions does not rule out either condition.

iii. Feline parvovirosis is usually diagnosed in shelter cats based on a combination of history (incomplete vaccination), clinical signs, results of fecal parvovirus antigen testing, and white blood cell count. Bacterial culture for *Salmonella* spp. may be performed, although demonstration of the bacterium in feces does not prove it is the cause; subclinical carriage is possible. If a cat dies or is euthanized, histopathology and immunohistochemistry provide a definitive diagnosis.

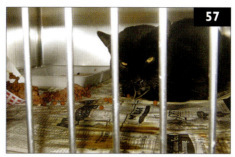

57 Case **57** is the same cat as case **56**. Concurrently, two other adult cats (57) in the same ward of the shelter became ill. Feces from both cats tested strongly positive on fecal tests for parvovirus antigen, and a blood smear showed few white blood cells in one of the cats. Feline parvovirosis was diagnosed. Both cats were euthanized, as adequate isolation and treatment facilities were not available. There were 25 other cats in the ward, ranging from 8 weeks of age to adult. All had received inactivated FPV, FHV, and FCV vaccines on intake and had been in the shelter for between 1 and 35 days. The cages were cleaned daily with a quaternary ammonium disinfectant.
i. How should the cages in which the two sick cats were be decontaminated?
ii. What should be recommended regarding the 25 exposed cats to prevent continued spread of this infection?

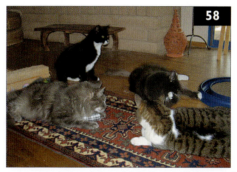

58 Case **58** is the same cat as cases **56** and **57**. Four of the adult cats in the shelter entered with a history of complete vaccination. They were clinically normal (58).
i. How high is the risk in these four cats of getting the disease?
ii. What vaccination protocol should be recommended in the future to reduce the risk of feline parvoviral outbreaks in this shelter?

57 i. Quaternary ammonium disinfectants do not inactivate FPV. The cages should be cleaned with detergent and water, then disinfected with a proven parvocide. Disinfectant should be left for a minimum of 10 minutes, and the cages allowed to dry thoroughly. If not inactivated or removed, parvoviruses can persist for many months.

ii. Exposed cats should be separated. If possible, they should be quarantined for 14 days. If not, the outbreak may continue unless they are euthanized. In shelters where a parvocidal disinfectant is used routinely and there is minimal fomite transmission, exposure may not occur. However, here, there is evidence that spread has already occurred; therefore, all cats in the ward should be considered exposed. This may occur up to 3 days before clinical signs are recognized. The risk of disease can be assessed as follows: (1) *Very low risk:* cats older than 4 months that have been given either a MLV vaccine or a series of two inactivated vaccines completed at least 1 week before exposure, and clinically normal cats with documented protective titers against FPV. (2) *Moderate risk:* kittens less than 4 months, even if appropriately vaccinated. (3) *High risk:* cats vaccinated only once with a MLV vaccine less than 1 week before exposure, cats vaccinated with a single inactivated vaccine at any time, or cats only vaccinated with IN vaccines. (4) *Highest risk:* all unvaccinated cats.

58 i. These four adult cats are not at significant risk. No special precautions need to be taken.

ii. Correct use of vaccines greatly reduces the risk of FPV spread in a shelter or other multiple-cat environment. Due to its rapid onset of protection, MLV vaccine is strongly recommended. Cats should be vaccinated immediately on intake to the shelter. Kittens should be vaccinated at 4–6 weeks of age; this should be repeated every 2–3 weeks as long as the kitten is in the shelter, until 16 weeks of age. Adult cats should be vaccinated once immediately on intake, and may be revaccinated after 2 weeks, particularly if there is any concern that the cat was ill at the time of the first vaccination. However, for pregnant cats, the risk of fetal damage from the vaccine should be weighed against the risk to queen and offspring of infection. Cats that cannot be vaccinated with a MLV vaccine for legal or medical reasons should be housed in a clean, isolated area, preferably outside the shelter.

59 A 7-year-old castrated male domestic shorthair cat was seen because of nasal discharge, sneezing, and a subcutaneous swelling on the forehead of 4 months' duration. The cat lived near Sydney, Australia. The disease had been unresponsive to treatment with antibiotics and corticosteroids. On examination, there was stertorous and frequently open-mouth breathing, absence of air

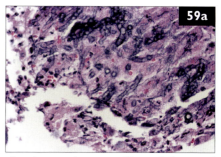

movement through the right nostril and a hard, prominent swelling of the nasal bridge. Slight bilateral nasal discharge was evident, and the mandibular lymph nodes were enlarged. Multiple pinch biopsies were obtained from the right side of the nasal cavity. Also, abnormal subcutaneous tissue was obtained from the swollen nasal bridge for histology (**59a**) and culture. This consisted of 'veins' of brown marbled tissue interspersed with off-white fibrous tissue.
i. What can be seen on the histologic sections?
ii. What is the diagnosis?
iii. How should this cat be treated?

60 An approximately 2-year-old spayed female domestic shorthair cat was evaluated for acute collapse and respiratory distress (**60**). The cat was a stray in Florida, USA, rescued 2 months previously; it had been kept exclusively indoors since then. The cat appeared to be healthy at the time of rescue, was negative on FeLV and FIV tests, and was vaccinated against FPV, FHV, FCV,

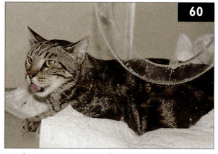

FeLV and rabies. On physical examination, the cat was vocalizing and appeared disoriented, was in severe respiratory distress, and was passing copious amounts of urine and bloody feces. There were increased bronchial sounds, so the heart sounds could not be heard. The mucous membranes were pale and cyanotic, the body temperature was decreased (37.2°C), the respiratory rate (65 bpm) was increased, and the pulse was not palpable.
i. What is the current condition of the cat?
ii. What immediate treatment and diagnostic procedures are indicated?

59 i. Biopsies from the nasal bridge mass were composed of masses of inflammatory cells, including plasma cells, eosinophils, and macrophages; and abundant necrotic material in which there were many fungal hyphae. The nasal pinch biopsies showed chronic inflammation, some epithelial and glandular hyperplasia, and a small number of fungal elements. Squash

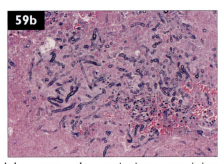

preparations of the excised brown material demonstrated necrotic tissue containing masses of hyphae (**59b**).

ii. Material from these sources was cultured on Sabouraud's glucose agar plates containing chloramphenicol and gentamicin. A filamentous fungus was isolated after 3 days' incubation at 28°C and identified as *Metarhizium anisopliae*. The cat was subsequently tested for FeLV and FIV, but it was negative for both. The diagnosis was, therefore, invasive rhinitis due to *Metarhizium anisopliae*.

iii. The cat was treated with itraconazole initially. After 2 weeks, the cat's breathing had improved, with better air movement through the right nostril. There was also reduction of sneezing and nasal discharge. After about 2 months, therapy was altered to ketoconazole for 80 days for financial reasons. Clinical signs of invasive mycotic rhinitis recurred 6 months after discontinuation of treatment, at which time the cat's owners were unprepared to pursue further therapy. Such a case would now be recommended posaconazole therapy (5 mg/kg once daily with food) as this drug has a greater spectrum of activity than itraconazole, is better tolerated, and is largely devoid of hepatic toxicity.

60 i. The cat is in acute hypotensive shock of unknown cause. Severe involvement of both the respiratory tract and the gastrointestinal tract suggests a systemic reaction such as anaphylaxis or electrocution, or a primary catastrophic gastrointestinal event. These all lead to respiratory failure, as the lung is the cat's shock organ. Trauma was considered to be unlikely in an indoor cat.

ii. Immediate treatment should include emergency supportive care and initial treatment for the most likely causes. Oxygen therapy and minimal handling were immediately employed to reduce stress. Furosemide and prednisolone were administered, and IV colloids were given to restore the circulating volume and blood pressure. Ampicillin/sublactam was administered IV due to the apparent disruption of the gastrointestinal mucosal barrier. Preparations were made for intubation and mechanical ventilation in case of deterioration. Specific diagnostic procedures were delayed pending stabilization of the patient.

61 Case 61 is the same cat as case 60. After 3 hours of emergency treatment, the cat was stable enough to begin diagnostic procedures.

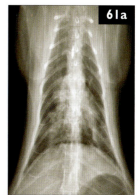

Blood profile/biochemistry panel	Results
Hematocrit – nonregenerative anemia	0.26 l/l
Neutrophilia	20.05 × 10⁹/l
Left shift band neutrophils	5.9 × 10⁹/l
Metamyelocytes	0.6 × 10⁹/l
Eosinophilia	2.3 × 10⁹/l
Basophilia	0.5 × 10⁹/l
Panhypoproteinemia	45 g/l
ALT – mild increase	203 IU/l

Lateral (**61a**) and ventrodorsal (**61b**) thoracic radiographs were taken.

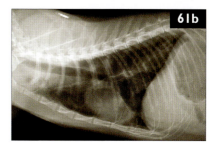

i. What is the assessment of the laboratory changes?
ii. What is the appearance of the thoracic radiographs?
iii. What diagnostic procedures should be performed next?

62 Case 62 is the same cat as cases 60 and 61. Abdominal radiographs and ultrasound examination were normal with the exception of a fluid-filled intestinal tract. The history of acute collapse with respiratory distress and the finding of eosinophilia were compatible with feline heartworm disease. A test for heartworm antibodies was negative, but a positive reaction was observed on a canine heartworm antigen test (**62a**). Several short segments of parallel lines were visualized in the area of the right ventricle on echocardiography (**62b**).

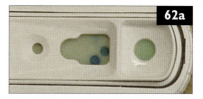

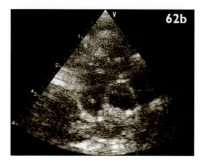

i. Are these results consistent with heartworm disease?
ii. Do these findings explain the clinical presentation of this cat?
iii. What treatment should be recommended?

61 i. These findings are consistent with a marked inflammatory reaction and the acute intestinal blood loss observed in this cat. The eosinophilia suggests possible parasitism or hypersensitivity reaction.
ii. The thoracic radiographs showed a patchy interstitial–alveolar pattern with enlargement of the caudal lobar pulmonary arteries.
iii. A complete blood count, biochemistry panel, urinalysis, clotting profile, fecal flotation, and repeat FeLV and FIV tests are indicated. Besides the thoracic radiographs, abdominal radiographs and abdominal ultrasound should also be performed.

62 i. The findings are diagnostic for feline heartworm disease (dirofilariasis). It is not uncommon for cats with heartworms to have negative heartworm antibody or antigen tests. The antigen tests detect parasite antigens, so tests developed for use in dogs may also be used in cats, but they are less sensitive in cats than in dogs due to the very low worm burden in cats. They are, however, highly specific, and a positive result indicates the presence of at least one adult female heartworm, or one that has recently died. Antibody tests are positive after exposure to larval or adult heartworms; however, they can also be false-negative in the cat.
ii. Although uncommon, anaphylaxis has been reported in heartworm-infected cats. Sudden death may occur, and is believed to be related to pulmonary reactions associated with a dying heartworm.
iii. Because of the high risk of patient death associated with a dying heartworm, adulticide therapy is contraindicated in cats. Clinical signs can often be managed medically with anti-inflammatory doses of corticosteroids and bronchodilators. Surgical treatment is indicated if medical therapy alone is inadequate. In this patient, a single heartworm was extracted *via* the jugular vein, and the cat was treated with doxycycline for 4 weeks.
    One year later, radiographs revealed the persistence of moderate broncho-interstitial disease, but the cat was clinically normal.

63 An 8-year-old spayed female Burmese cat was seen because of a 4-day history of vomiting and inappetence. On physical examination the cat was 10% dehydrated, had icteric mucous membranes, and a high body temperature (40.1°C). Ultrasonography (63), complete blood count, biochemistry panel, and urinalysis were performed (1 – gall bladder; 2 – sludge). The significant results were:

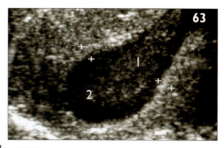

Blood profile/biochemistry panel	Results
White blood cells	$3.7 \times 10^9/l$
Mature neutrophils	$0.10 \times 10^9/l$
Band neutrophils	$1.90 \times 10^9/l$
Lymphocytes	$0.90 \times 10^9/l$
ALT	428 IU/l
ALP	9 IU/l
Total protein	82 g/l
Albumin	26 g/l
Globulins	56 g/l
Bilirubin	33 µmol/l
Creatinine	260 µmol/l
Urea	25 mmol/l
Urinalysis	
Specific gravity	1.052; all normal

i. How can the laboratory results be interpreted?
ii. What does the ultrasonography show?
iii. What should be done next?

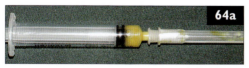

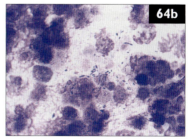

64 Case 64 is the same cat as in case 63. An aspirate from the gall bladder (64a) was collected, and a cytologic preparation of the aspirate (64b) (modified Wrights–Giemsa) was prepared.
i. What are the findings in the aspirate cytology?
ii. What is the etiopathogenesis of acute cholangitis in cats?

63 i. There is a neutropenia with a very low number of segmented neutrophils and a high number of band neutrophils (left shift) and a lymphopenia. This may reflect marked inflammatory demand. A less likely explanation is immune-mediated destruction of mature neutrophils. Lymphopenia may be due to endogenous corticosteroid production in acute inflammatory disease, viral infections (e.g. FeLV, FIV) or from increased loss (e.g. intestinal disease). The cat was tested for FeLV antigen and FIV antibody and was FIV-positive. Hyperbilirubinemia indicates cholestasis. Hemolysis as a prehepatic cause of hyperbilirubinemia can be ruled out because the cat is not anemic. Therefore, the mechanisms of cholestasis are hepatic or posthepatic. There is evidence of hepatocellular necrosis (elevated ALT activity). It is not unusual to see normal activities of ALP in icteric cats since the half-life of ALP in cats is less than 6 hours. Dehydration is reflected by prerenal azotemia.

ii. On ultrasonography the gall-bladder wall appears thickened and hyperechoic, suggesting inflammation or edema. The bile within the gall bladder is hyperechoic. While this can be a normal finding in cats, it may indicate inspissation or suppuration of the bile.

iii. A bile aspirate is indicated. The most expedient method is by percutaneous, ultrasound-guided cholecystocentesis. The sample should be submitted for cytologic examination and culture.

64 i. The gall bladder contents are yellow in contrast to the normal dark green color of bile, suggestive of suppurative infection. Bile from healthy cats is sterile. The modified Wrights–Giemsa stain reveals the presence of bacterial bacilli among a background of degenerate cells. On Gram stain the bacilli found in this cat were Gram-negative and a pure culture of *Salmonella enterica* serovar *typhimurium* was isolated from bile.

ii. The anatomy of the feline biliary tract is unique. The common bile duct and pancreatic duct enter the duodenum together at the major duodenal papilla. Compared to dogs and humans, cats have very high numbers of bacteria in their proximal small intestine including obligate and facultative anerobes. Abnormalities in intestinal motility may allow reflux of intestinal contents into the common bile duct and secondary bacterial colonization. In pancreatitis, reflux of pancreatic ductal contents into the common bile duct may cause transient cholestasis and also enable bacterial colonization and infection. Thus triaditis, the combination of cholangitis, pancreatitis, and IBD, may be seen in some cats. Most cases of acute cholangitis are associated with mixed infections of anerobes and aerobes, such as *Escherichia coli*, *Clostridia* spp., *Fusobacterium* spp., *Actinomyces* spp., *Streptococcus* spp., and *Bacteroides* spp., all members of normal intestinal flora. *Salmonella* spp. have been isolated with a frequency of 1–18% from the feces of healthy cats.

65 A 9-year-old spayed female Burmese cat from the USA died suddenly in front of the owners. The cat had a history of asthma that was periodically treated with prednisolone. There were two related Burmese cats in the home that appeared to be healthy. All cats were current on vaccinations and were kept inside. The body was presented for necropsy, which was unremark- able with the exception of congested lungs (65a) (H&E stain).

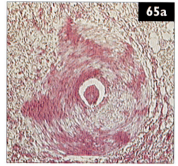

i. What does this histologic section reveal?
ii. Are the other cats in the household at risk from the same disease?

66 A 3-year-old spayed female domestic shorthair cat (66a) was referred for chronic hematuria and dysuria unresponsive to antibio- tics. The cat, which was otherwise healthy, was kept indoors with one other healthy cat. It was fed dry food for cats with urinary disease. Physical examination was normal. Abdominal radiographs showed that both kidneys were normal and showed no uroliths in the bladder, and a small bladder with a thickened wall was seen on ultrasonography (66b). Urinalysis and urine culture were performed; urine culture was negative. Urinalysis of a cystocentesis sample showed the following abnormalities:

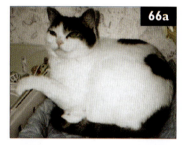

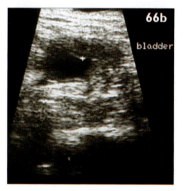

Urinalysis	Results
Color, appearance	yellow, cloudy
Protein	(+)
Blood	++++
RBC	10–50 cells/hpf
WBC	5–10 cells/hpf

i. How is this cat's problem defined?
ii. What are the differential diagnoses?
iii. What further tests should be performed?
iv. How should the cat be treated?

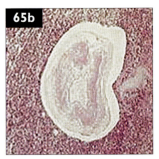
65b

65 i. The most prominent finding is the markedly hypertrophied wall of the pulmonary arteriole. There is inflammation of the interstitial tissues and a thrombus in the lumen of the arteriole. This pulmonary arteriolar occlusive hypertrophy with interstitial inflammation is a classic manifestation of feline heartworm-associated respiratory disease (HARD), which can develop in the presence of either larval or adult heartworm life stages. The pulmonary changes and associated 'asthma-like' clinical signs of coughing and respiratory distress may persist even after the parasites are eliminated. An additional lung section revealed a dead heartworm cut in cross-section in a pulmonary arteriole (65b). In this case, the arteriolar wall was deteriorating, and there was marked adjacent inflammation obliterating the alveoli. Sudden death is one of the most common signs of heartworm infection in cats.

ii. Heartworm-infected cats are rarely microfilaremic, so they are considered to be dead-end hosts for *Dirofilaria immitis*. Even though the infected cat does not pose a threat of transmission to the other cats, all the cats in the household share similar risks for exposure to mosquitoes bearing infectious *Dirofilaria immitis* L3 larvae. Heartworm-preventive medication should be recommended for all cats living in regions where dirofilariasis is endemic in dogs. Indoor lifestyle does not protect cats against heartworm infection.

66 i. The presenting problem is inappropriate urination with hematuria and dysuria. The urinalysis indicates microscopic hematuria with mild pyuria. These findings are compatible with lower urinary tract disease.

ii. The major causes of lower urinary tract signs without urethral obstruction in young adult cats are: (1) idiopathic cystitis, and (2) bladder uroliths.

Bladder uroliths are unlikely in this case, as most uroliths in the bladder of cats are radio-opaque and are evident only on good quality abdominal radiographs.

iii. Cystoscopy with biopsy could also be performed. Cystitis in the cat is usually sterile; the causes remain unknown. Therefore, antibiotics should not be used in young cats. Bacterial cystitis is more common in cats older than 10 years of age. Voided samples should not be used for diagnosis, since these samples can be contaminated by normal flora bacteria. Instead, a cystocentesis sample should be obtained. Administration of a diuretic, sedative, or analgesic may be needed. Ultrasound guidance can also help.

iv. The diet should be changed to canned foods; these are beneficial due to their higher water content. Should this prove ineffective, other therapies, such as pain control or amitriptyline, could be considered.

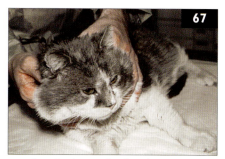

67 A 12-year-old castrated male domestic shorthair cat was seen because of slight lethargy and a rough hair coat (67). It had tested FIV-positive 2 years ago, but had remained healthy. It was an indoor-only cat in a single-cat household. Physical examination revealed a rough hair coat, slightly enlarged mandibular and popliteal lymph nodes, and severe stomatitis. Complete blood count showed leukopenia (3.5×10^9/l) due to a marked neutropenia (mature neutrophils 0.8×10^9/l) without a left shift (band neutrophils 0×10^9/l). Otherwise, the complete blood count, biochemical panel, and urinalysis were normal.
i. How should the neutropenia be treated in an FIV-infected cat?
ii. Should a neutropenic FIV-infected cat be treated with antibiotics?
iii. Should immune stimulators be used in this cat?

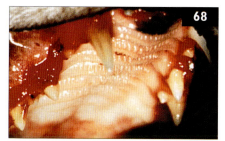

68 Case 68 is the same cat as case 67. Besides the rough hair coat, the cat had slightly enlarged mandibular and popliteal lymph nodes, and a severe stomatitis (68).
i. Which antiviral drug could be used in this cat?
ii. Are interferons useful in FIV-infected cats?
iii. What can be done to treat the stomatitis in this cat?

67 i. Some researchers have used cytokines to treat the neutropenia, but filgastrim is contraindicated in FIV-infected cats. Although it increases neutrophil counts in cats with FIV infection, all develop a significant increase in FIV virus load. Erythropoietin (human recombinant) is used in cats with nonregenerative anemia secondary to chronic renal failure. In contrast to treatment with filgastrim, no increased virus loads were observed in one study, and a gradual increase in white blood cell counts was also seen. Thus, erythropoietin can be used safely in FIV-infected cats.

ii. The answer to this question is controversial. It is likely that the FIV infection is responsible for the neutropenia in this cat, and cats with severe neutropenia are more susceptible to secondary bacterial infections. If no antibiotics are given, this cat should be monitored very closely; if the body temperature rises, a secondary bacterial infection could be present, and should be treated as soon as possible.

iii. 'Immune stimulators' or 'immune modulators' are widely used medications in FIV-infected cats. These restore compromised immune function; there is, however, no evidence that they have any beneficial effects on the health or survival of either asymptomatic or symptomatic FIV-infected cats. Nonspecific stimulation of the immune system might even be contraindicated, because it may cause increased virus replication. Thus, nonspecific immunomodulators with unknown effects should not be used in FIV-infected cats.

68 i. Some human antivirals can be used to treat FIV infection. AZT (zidovudine) has some effect in FIV-infected cats, especially in cats with stomatitis or neurologic signs. It improves quality of life and prolongs life expectancy. During treatment, complete blood counts should be performed regularly because nonregenerative anemia is a common side-effect. Thus, cats with bone marrow suppression should not be treated. Unfortunately, AZT-resistant mutants of FIV can arise as early as after 6 months of treatment.

ii. Human interferon-α is used commonly in cats. When given SC, it becomes ineffective after 3–7 weeks due to the development of neutralizing antibodies. If given PO, it is not absorbed but destroyed in the gastrointestinal tract, and it has only immunomodulatory effects by stimulating the lymphoid tissue in the oral cavity. Feline interferon-ω was recently licensed in some European countries and Japan. It can be used long-term without antibody development. No side-effects have been reported in cats, and it is active against FIV *in vitro*. So far, only one study has been performed with feline interferon-ω, in which it did not show significant changes in survival rate.

iii. In this cat, full-mouth dental extraction was performed, and the stomatitis improved significantly.

69 A 3-year-old spayed female domestic shorthair cat was seen because of a solid pinkish-white mass in the left eye (69). The pupil was misshapen and did not dilate or constrict normally. The cat was otherwise healthy. It was kept indoors only, and was current on all vaccinations. Slit lamp examination of the left anterior chamber revealed a small amount of flare. The solid pinkish mass

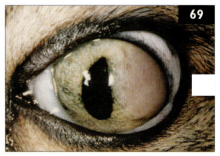

arose from the iris and bulged into the anterior chamber. There were fine vessels on the surface of the iris, which was diffusely swollen. The lens was normal, as were the vitreous and retina in both eyes. A full ophthalmic examination was performed; the significant results were:

Ophthalmic examination	Right eye (OD)	Left eye (OS)
PLR	+	slow and incomplete
(direct and indirect)		
IOP	17 mmHg	10 mmHg

i. What is the ocular diagnosis and what are the differential diagnoses?
ii. What diagnostic tests are indicated?
iii. Is the misshapen pupil significant?

70 A 3-year-old castrated male domestic shorthair cat was seen because of multifocal alopecia (70) that was first noticed 2 months ago. Initially, the alopecic areas were barely noticeable, but they increased in size with time, and moderate scaling of the affected skin was also noticed. No crusts or papules were observed. The cat was vaccinated

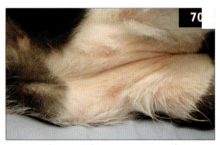

and regularly wormed, and had free access to outdoors. There were no other pets in the household. Physical examination showed no abnormalities other than dermatologic changes. Multifocal alopecia with mild to moderate fine scaling was noted on the hocks.
i. What are the differential diagnoses for this cat?
ii. What should the diagnostic approach be?

69 i. There is a mass and flare in the anterior chamber of the left eye, and a low IOP. These symptoms indicate anterior uveitis, probably due to a neoplasm. Possible etiologies of uveitis in the cat include infectious diseases, neoplasia (e.g. lymphoma), and immune-mediated diseases.

ii. The lesion in the anterior chamber is associated with the anterior uveal tract. An ocular ultrasound examination is indicated to evaluate the size and dimensions of the mass, which could extend posteriorly into the vitreous. Because ocular neoplasia is strongly suspected, further diagnostic tests should include a complete blood count, biochemistry panel, urinalysis, and FIP, FeLV, and FIV tests. Additional tests should include thoracic and abdominal radiographs, abdominal ultrasound, and lymph node and/or bone marrow aspirates. Complete blood count revealed mild nonregenerative anemia. Antigen testing for FeLV was positive. Cytologic examination of bone marrow aspirates confirmed the diagnosis of lymphoma, which is the most frequent intraocular tumor in cats.

iii. Changes of the contour of the iris may indicate uveal and irideal infiltration with neoplastic lesions or posterior synechiae in chronic cases of uveitis. In cats, a 'D-shaped' or 'reverse D-shaped' pupil may be seen. This is caused by damage to the ciliary innervation and results in functional deficits of the pupil. A D-shaped pupil may be observed in FeLV-infected cats without any other clinical symptoms.

70 i. Multifocal alopecia in the cat may be due to: (1) Self-trauma. (2) Inflammation of the hair follicle (e.g. with dermatophytosis, demodicosis, and bacterial pyoderma). (3) Damage to the hair shaft with subsequent breakage (e.g. with dermatophytosis). (4) Destruction of the hair follicle (e.g. with immune-mediated alopecia areata). (5) Lack of regrowth (e.g. with very rare hormonal diseases).

ii. Firstly, it should be established whether the skin is pruritic or non-pruritic. However, this may be hard to ascertain, as some cats do not lick in front of their owner. If pruritic, allergic diseases (e.g. fleas, food, or environmental allergens) or psychogenic causes are most likely. If nonpruritic, the hairs in the affected area should be examined to see whether the hair tips are broken off, or are tapered, as in hormonal disease. If broken off, examination under a Wood's lamp for fluorescence of hair shafts infected with dermatophytes is indicated. However, false-positive and false-negative results are common – many dermatophytes (including 50% of *M. canis*) do not fluoresce. If this test is negative, a dermatophyte culture is indicated, using hair and scales from the edges of the lesions. A deep skin scraping is also needed to rule out the rare feline demodicosis. If all these tests are negative, allergic disease should be considered. Also, taking a biopsy is helpful to rule out unusual causes of multifocal alopecia.

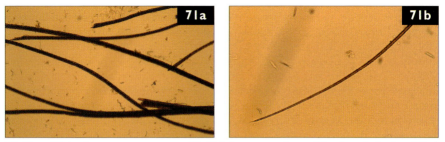

71 Case 71 is the same cat as case 70. Trichograms showed broken hair tips (71a) in comparison to normal hair (71b), Wood's lamp examination was negative, and fungal culture revealed *Microsporum canis*.
i. What are the treatment options for dermatophytosis?
ii. For how long should the cat be treated?

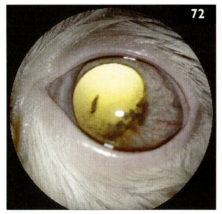

72 A 4-year-old castrated male domestic shorthair cat was seen because of an ocular abnormality first noticed by the client 2 days previously. On physical examination, the left eye had white keratic precipitates in the anterior chamber and aqueous flare (72). The IOP of the affected eye was subnormal at 12 mmHg compared to that of the right eye at 18 mmHg. No abnormalities were seen on fundic examination.
i. What are the differential diagnoses for anterior uveitis?
ii. How is a diagnosis of *Toxoplasma gondii*-induced uveitis made?
iii. What are the risks to the cat if untreated?

71 i. Treatment options include topical therapy, systemic therapy, or a combination thereof. Failure to use sporicidal topical therapy allows further environmental contamination with spore- laden hair shafts. Because fungal spores have been cultured up to 2–3 inches (1–1.5 cm) away from lesions, whole-body treatments such as rinses with enilconazole or lyme sulfur are required. Owners need to be educated about the zoonotic potential of *M. canis* (especially in immunosuppressed people and small children). If there is increased concern about transmission of the infection to humans or in severe cases, additional systemic antifungal therapy may be considered. Griseofulvin, itraconazole, or terbinafine may all be useful. Griseofulvin may cause bone marrow suppression in some cats, particularly those infected with FIV, and weekly blood counts for the first month should be recommended. Griseofulvin is also teratogenic and should not be used in pregnant cats. Itraconazole may occasionally be hepatotoxic, although increased liver enzyme activity is usually not an indication to stop therapy unless clinical signs also occur.
ii. Treatment should be extended for at least 1–2 months beyond clinical remission and negative fungal cultures.

72 i. FIP, bartonellosis, toxoplasmosis, systemic mycoses, and infection with FeLV, FIV, or FHV are the main infectious differential diagnoses.
ii. Demonstration of increasing *T. gondii* IgM antibody titers in paired samples is indicative of acute or reactivated infection. As *T. gondii* cysts remain lifelong, long-term antibody titers are expected, and do not necessarily represent active infection. Antibody concentrations in aqueous humor fluid may also be measured. To ensure that the aqueous humor antibodies have not diffused across damaged vascular barriers, a comparison of serum and aqueous antibody levels for *T. gondii* and a nonocular infectious agent, such as calicivirus, is used. In this case, the ratio of *T. gondii* antibodies to calicivirus antibodies was higher in the aqueous humor than in the blood. Furthermore, no antibodies to other infections were found in the aqueous humor, making the diagnosis of toxoplasmosis very likely.
iii. If anterior uveitis is not treated, the resultant inflammation may lead to lens luxation, glaucoma, retinal detachment, and blindness. The recommended therapeutic protocol for toxoplasmal uveitis consists of clindamycin given orally for 4 weeks, and a short course of topical ophthalmic glucocorticoids. In this cat, after 3 weeks of treatment, the left anterior chamber precipitates were nearly resolved and the IOP returned to 18 mmHg in both eyes. Therapy was continued for 3 more weeks, at which time the eyes and IOP appeared normal.

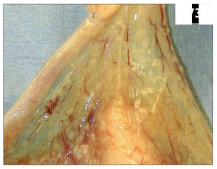

73 An 8-month-old intact female domestic shorthair cat was seen for elective ovariohysterectomy. The owner had obtained the cat and its male littermate at the age of 8 weeks from a neighbor. Both kittens grew normally and had received two vaccinations against FPV, FHV, and FCV. FeLV and FIV tests were negative. Physical examination was unremarkable. At the beginning of the surgery, the left uterine horn was elevated through a 2-cm midline abdominal incision. It was noted that the broad ligament, which is usually transparent in cats, was opacified by an off-white nodular infiltrate. Similar 2–4 mm nodules were present on the uterine horn and ovary. There was a slightly icteric hue to the tissues (73).

i. What are the differential diagnoses for the condition?
ii. What is the best immediate course of action?

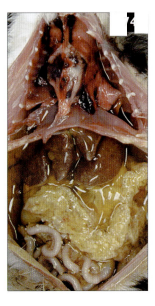

74 Case 74 is the same cat as case 73. Following the finding of an abnormal uterus and ovary during routine ovariohysterectomy, the incision was extended to permit thorough exploration of the abdomen. Multifocal serosal nodules were present on all serosal surfaces, including the organs, diaphragm, and body wall. The omentum had formed a tight clump and was stained yellow. A moderate amount of clear yellow peritoneal effusion was present. Cytologic evaluation of the fluid revealed a high-protein modified transudate containing nondegenerate neutrophils and macrophages, and the Rivalta test was positive. No organisms were seen on cytology. The owner was contacted and elected euthanasia without recovering the cat from anesthesia. A necropsy was performed and revealed effusions of the peritoneal, pleural, and pericardial cavities (74). Histologic evaluation revealed pyogranulomatous inflammation and neutrophilic vasculitis.

i. What is the diagnosis?
ii. What is the prognosis for the littermate of this cat?

73 i. Infiltrative conditions in the abdomen of cats include inflammatory diseases (e.g. FIP, other granulomatous diseases, steatitis, peritonitis, pancreatitis), mineralization, and abnormal adipose accumulation. In most cases, clinical signs would be expected to accompany these conditions.

ii. At the time of surgery, the most appropriate action would be to extend the incision to examine the abdomen more thoroughly. The owner should be contacted to be appraised of the findings and for permission to perform any additional invasive procedures such as biopsies.

74 i. The clinical findings and histopathologic results are most consistent with FIP. Although the cat had no apparent clinical signs, the disease process was well-developed, and the cat would have been expected to develop typical signs soon. Once clinical signs develop, deterioration and death usually occur in weeks to months.

ii. Minimally pathogenic enteric FCoV are widespread. For reasons that are not fully understood, they sometimes mutate, making them capable of systemic circulation. FIP is believed to arise as an immune-mediated response to systemic infection with FCoV. The genetic background of individual cats plays a role here. Also, kittens and young adults appear to be more susceptible to disease development than older cats. It is likely that the littermate was also exposed to and infected with FCoV, and since it shares some genetic similarities with the affected cat, there may be an increased risk that it, too, will develop FIP. However, most cats that are exposed to coronavirus do not develop FIP. The littermate should receive good preventive health care and diet to promote a healthy immune system. Elective surgeries and stressful events should be avoided at this time as these have been associated with exacerbations of FIP.

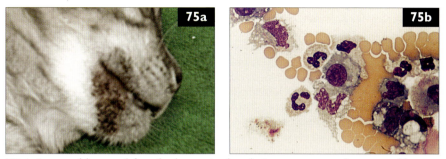

75 A 3-year-old spayed female domestic shorthair cat was seen because of bumps and scabs on its chin. The cat lived with four other cats, two of which also had similar lesions. On physical examination, the entire chin and perioral regions were affected (75a). Comedones and pustules were present along with black casts in the fur. The lesions did not appear to bother the cat. Cytologic examination of pustular contents was performed (75b).
i. What are the differential diagnoses for this condition?
ii. How is the diagnosis made?
iii. How is this disease treated?

76 A 1-year-old neutered male domestic shorthair cat was seen because of a 10-day history of ataxia (76). The cat was allowed access to both indoors and outdoors. It had been vaccinated twice against FPV, FHV, and FCV. Recently, the cat had been lethargic and had developed a head tilt and progressive bilateral pelvic limb ataxia. The body temperature was 40.4°C, the heart rate

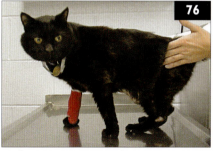

was 200 bpm, and the respiratory rate was 30 bpm. Mucous membranes were pale, and the mandibular lymph nodes were slightly enlarged. Neurologic examination showed reduced mental status, mild head tilt to the left, and severe pelvic limb ataxia. Postural reactions were reduced in both pelvic limbs and the left thoracic limb. Spinal reflexes and cranial nerve examinations were normal, except for the presence of positional vertical nystagmus.
i. What is the neuroanatomical localization of the neurologic signs?
ii. What are the likely differential diagnoses?

75 i. Acne, demodicosis, *Malassezia* spp. dermatitis, plastic contact hypersensitivity, and dermatophytosis are the major differential diagnoses.

ii. Cytologic examination of pustular contents shows intracellular and extracellular bacteria, degenerating neutrophils, and macrophages. Histopathologic evaluation of skin biopsies detected dilated, keratin-filled follicles, folliculitis, furunculosis, and fibrosis in this case, which is consistent with a diagnosis of feline acne.

iii. Cleansing with a 2% benzoyl peroxide shampoo or an antimicrobial cleanser (rinsing the skin well after use in both cases) is a critical part of the treatment of feline acne. A 2% mupirocin gel applied twice daily for 3–6 weeks may also be considered. Clindamycin may be effective as part of the therapeutic regime and should be continued for 1 week beyond clinical resolution. Retinoids can be used cautiously, monitoring for potential side-effects, including elevation in liver enzyme activities, irritation, pruritus, dry mucous membranes, and conjunctivitis.

76 i. Head tilt indicates vestibular disease, which can be either peripheral (inner ear, vestibulocochlear nerve) or central (brainstem, vestibulocerebellum). On neurologic examination, central vestibular disease is indicated by postural reaction deficits, vertical nystagmus, nystagmus with obvious changes in direction, or cranial nerve deficits other than facial paresis (VII) or Horner's syndrome. The facial nerve and sympathetic innervation of the eye can be affected by middle ear disease, but brainstem disease is also a possible cause. Proprioceptive positioning is considered the best test to distinguish peripheral from central vestibular disease, because ascending proprioceptive pathways are commonly disrupted with brainstem lesions, causing delayed postural reactions. Contrary to dogs, hopping or wheelbarrowing may be more sensitive for the recognition of postural reaction deficits in cats than conscious proprioceptive positioning. In the present case, central vestibular (brainstem) disease was diagnosed because of vertical nystagmus and decreased postural reactions.

ii. The main differentials for acute progressive brainstem disease in a cat of less than 1 year of age are inflammatory CNS disease (e.g. FIP, toxoplasmosis, bacterial encephalitis of hematogenous or otic origin, cryptococcosis, migrating *Cuterebra* larvae, polioencephalomyelitis, viral encephalitis); nutritional causes (e.g. thiamine deficiency); toxic causes (e.g. metronidazole, chlorinated hydrocarbons); or hereditary neurodegenerative disorders. Also, lymphoma always remains a possibility in cats that test positive for FeLV.

77 Case 77 is the same cat as case 76. In addition to the neurologic signs, there was gross hemorrhage and cloudiness within the anterior chamber of the left eye (77).
i. What are the likely differential diagnoses for the ophthalmic findings?
ii. What diagnostic procedures should be performed?
iii. Can the probable diagnosis be confirmed?

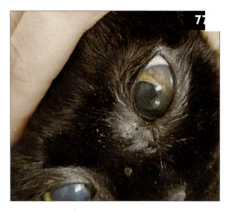

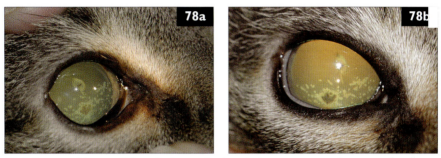

78 A 1-year-old spayed female domestic shorthair cat was seen because of redness, squinting, tearing, and speckling of the cornea in the right eye for a few days. The cat had recently been obtained from a shelter. It had outdoor access, was current on all vaccinations, and was regularly wormed. Recent FeLV and FIV testing was negative. The cat appeared normal apart from the right eye. There were multiple keratic precipitates attached to the inside of the cornea (78a), and there was mild to moderate flare in the anterior chamber (78b). The iris was hyperemic, and the vitreous had moderate cellular infiltration. A complete blood count, biochemistry panel, and urinalysis were performed. These showed anemia, neutrophilia with a left shift, lymphopenia, hyperbilirubinemia, and elevated total proteins with a decreased A:G ratio in the blood tests.
i. What are keratic precipitates, and what is their significance?
ii. What is the probable etiology of the ocular lesions?
iii. What additional diagnostic tests should be performed?
iv. What treatment is recommended for the right eye?

77 i. The ophthalmic findings are indicative of anterior uveitis. FIP is commonly associated with anterior uveitis and hemorrhagic exudates in the anterior chamber. However, other causes include fungal diseases, toxoplasmosis, FeLV infection, bartonellosis, and, less commonly, bacterial sepsis and coagulation disorders. FIP is often associated with fever and is a frequent cause of progressive neurologic disease in young cats.

ii. CSF analysis is the method of choice to diagnose the cause of CNS inflammation. Cytology is useful; increased leukocyte numbers are indicative of inflammation. In this case, a small amount of CSF with a high fibrin content and yellow color was collected. This had high leukocyte (mainly neutrophil) and protein counts. No organisms were seen. These findings are suspicious of FIP. Otoscopic examination should have ruled out ear disease. A complete blood count, biochemical profile, and urinalysis should also be evaluated. Ultrasonography of the abdomen should be performed to look for effusions or granulomatous infiltrates.

iii. FIP meningoencephalitis is very hard to diagnose. Currently, PCR tests do not distintinguish between 'harmless' enteric FCoV and FIP-causing viruses. Thus, a positive PCR result cannot provide proof for the diagnosis of CNS FIP. Extraneural FIP can be diagnosed by biopsy of affected tissues. Positive immunohistochemical staining of biopsy specimens or cytologic preparations from effusions provides definitive proof for the diagnosis of FIP.

78 i. Keratic precipitates are accumulations of cellular debris (e.g. macrophages, mononuclear cells) on the endothelium of the cornea. They can be very finely granular in appearance or may coalesce to larger deposits. They are a typical sign of anterior uveitis and are considered pathognomonic for granulomatous-type inflammation.

ii. The ocular findings, together with the laboratory results, are highly suggestive of an infectious cause of the ocular lesions, particularly FIP. Ocular lesions are seen with all forms of systemic FIP or may be present in an otherwise asymptomatic cat. However, they are not diagnostic for FIP; similar lesions may be seen with FeLV or FIV infection.

iii. Thoracic and abdominal radiographs, abdominal ultrasound, liver biopsy, and aqueous centesis can be performed for final diagnosis of FIP infection. Also, FIP can be positively diagnosed by the Rivalta test, in which immunohistochemical staining shows FCoV-antigen in macrophages in a body cavity effusion or biopsies from organs.

iv. This should include a potent anti-inflammatory drug. The treatment of choice for anterior uveitis in cats is topical prednisolone acetate. If a corneal ulcer is detected, topical nonsteroidal anti-inflammatory drugs, such as flurbiprofen or diclofenac, are suitable alternatives. In addition, topical atropine ointment should be applied for pupillary dilation, stabilization of the blood–aqueous barrier, and control of pain.

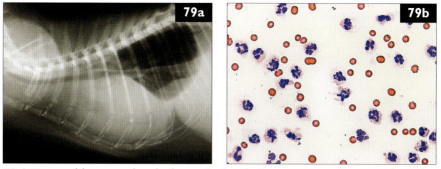

79 A 7-year-old castrated male domestic shorthair cat was seen because of a 3-day history of lethargy and anorexia. The owner had noted labored breathing for several days. The cat was current on vaccinations and was an indoor/outdoor cat with two other cats living in the same household. On physical examination, the patient had a high respiratory rate and dull heart and lung sounds. The patient was febrile and slightly dehydrated. Thoracic radiographs (79a) showed effusion in both pleural cavities. The complete blood count demonstrated neutrophilia with a left shift; serum biochemistry panel and urinalysis were unremarkable. Thoracocentesis, fluid analysis, and cytologic examination of the fluid (79b) were performed. The most significant findings of the fluid analysis were specific gravity 1.038, white blood cells 237 × 10⁹/l, total protein 66 g/l, LDH 3005 IU/l, α-Amylase 1658 IU/l, triglycerides 0.4 mmol/l.
i. What is the diagnosis?
ii. What can cause this disease?

80 Case 80 is the same cat as case 79. In the bacterial culture, growth of *Nocardia asteroides* was identified (80).
i. What other diagnostic tests should be performed?
ii. How should the cat be treated?

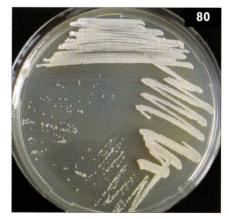

79 i. The diagnosis in this cat is pyothorax. Pyothorax is a septic inflammation of the pleural cavity. Typical for this type of effusion is the high leukocyte count ($>5 \times 10^9$ cells/l), the high protein content (>33 g/l), the high specific gravity (>1.030), and a significant number of neutrophils, often characterized by extensive degranulation on cytology. Intracellular bacteria can be observed on cytology.
ii. Possible etiologies of pyothorax are migrating foreign bodies, bite wounds, penetrating thoracic wounds, extension from pneumonia, esophageal perforation, extensions of cervical, lumbar or mediastinal infections, or hematogenous spread leading to bacterial contamination and infection of the pleural cavity. In this patient from a multi-cat household and with access to the outdoors, a penetrating bite wound or a migrating foreign body could be likely explanations, although spread of infection from other locations in the body can certainly not be excluded. Bacteria isolated most frequently from cats with pyothorax are *Pasteurella multocida* and anerobic bacterial species. Less frequently isolated organisms include *Nocardia asteroides*, *Actimomyces* spp., and many other aerobic Gram-positive and Gram-negative bacteria. Rarely, fungal organisms, such as *Aspergillus* spp. and *Cryptococcus neoformans*, have been cultured from cases of feline pyothorax.

80 i. Ultrasonography of the pleural cavity should be performed to look for possible encapsulated areas, abscesses, or masses in the lungs or mediastinum. Intrathoracic structures can be evaluated better while fluid is still present. If masses are found, fine-needle aspirates can be taken for cytology with ultrasound guidance. Then, the pleural cavity should be drained, and new thoracic radiographs should be taken. Also, culture and sensitivity testing of the pleural fluid should be performed.
ii. Treatment of pyothorax should be both medical and surgical. If there is a significant amount of septic pleural fluid, drainage is indicated. This can be continuous with a closed suction system, or intermittent, by syringe several times daily. Intermittent drainage is preferred if continuous monitoring of the patient is not possible. In addition, pleural lavage may be performed. The chest tubes can be removed when the thoracic effusion has significantly decreased and serial cytology of the effusion shows only low leukocyte counts and no bacteria.

In addition to surgical treatment, antibiotic therapy is given for at least 4–6 weeks, until clinical and radiological abnormalities have resolved. Broad-spectrum antibiotics are administered IV while results from culture and sensitivity testing are pending. In addition, fluid therapy and pain management are required. Sulfonamides are the initial treatment of choice for nocardiosis. However, not all isolates are sensitive to sulfonamides.

81 A 6-year-old spayed female Siamese cat was seen for respiratory distress. It had been treated with cyclosporin (6 mg/kg q 12 h PO for 8 weeks) for immune-mediated hemolytic anemia. On physical examination, the cat had a high body temperature (40.5°C) and was tachypneic (60 bpm) with increased inspiratory effort. Thoracic radiographs reveal bilateral pleural effusion. A cytologic preparation of a pleural fluid aspirate was made (81) (modified Wrights–Giemsa). Tests for FIV and FeLV were negative.

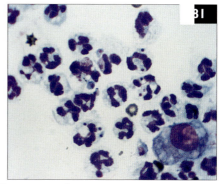

i. What are the findings in the cytology of the pleural fluid aspirate?
ii. What are the shortcomings of antibody tests in this disease?

82 A 1-year-old intact male domestic shorthair cat was seen because of a 6-month history of ulcerated and nodular lesions. The cat lived mainly outdoors. Initial treatment had consisted of one glucocorticoid injection followed by oral prednisone and amoxicillin; there had been no response. On physical examination, the cat was bright and alert. Multiple nodular and crusted lesions with occasional draining tracts and ulcerations of varying size were found on the bridge of the nose (82a), eyelids, ear margins, and front legs. A direct imprint from the bridge of the nose was examined microscopically after staining with modified Wright's stain. It showed degenerated neutrophils, few macrophages, and numerous round to oval yeast-like organisms (82b, arrow).

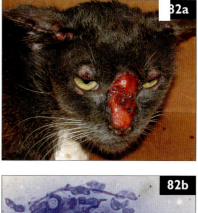

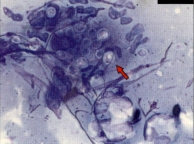

i. What are the differential diagnoses, and what is the tentative diagnosis?
ii. What is known about the etiology and pathogenesis?
iii. What other clinical signs may be present?
iv. What further tests will confirm the diagnosis?

81 i. In the cytologic preparation, there are many nondegenerate neutrophils, few red blood cells, and few macrophages. Within the cytoplasm of many of the neutrophils are protozoal tachyzoites with morphology suggestive of *Toxoplasma gondii*. The high dose of cyclosporin probably immunosuppressed the cat, resulting in reactivated toxoplasmosis.

ii. Detection of antibodies against *T. gondii* does not equate to clinical disease and cannot differentiate latent from active infections. Approximately 20% of cats fail to develop IgM titers, and positive IgM titers can persist months to years after infection. In reactivated toxoplasmosis no IgM response may occur. In FIV-positive cats, an IgM response may not occur or the class shift to IgG may be delayed. High IgG titers may persist for more than 6 years postinfection.

82 i. The tentative diagnosis is cutaneous sporotrichosis (infection with *Sporothrix schenkii*). Other differential diagnoses are deep bacterial infections (nocardiosis, atypical mycobacterial infection, actinomycosis, feline leprosy) or other fungal infections (histoplasmosis, cryptococcosis, blastomycosis, coccidiodomycosis, phaeohyphomycosis).

ii. *Sporothrix schenkii* is a worldwide, ubiquitous, saprophytic and dimorphic fungus. Most commonly, the infection occurs in outdoor cats due to puncture wounds from claws and bites and, sometimes, plants. In this cat, autoinoculation due to grooming and rubbing of the lesions probably contributed to the spreading of the skin lesions. Previous therapy with glucocorticoids may have contributed as well to the progression of the skin lesions.

iii. Other signs are lethargy, depression, anorexia, fever, and respiratory tract signs. A complete blood count and biochemistry profile often show anemia, leukocytosis with neutrophilia, hypoalbuminemia, and hyperglobulinemia.

iv. Cytologic and histopathologic examinations are effective in detecting the fungus, but to specify the organism, fungal cultures from exudates or skin tissue are necessary. The typical histopathologic findings are nodular to diffuse, pyogranulomatous dermatitis with intralesional yeast-like organisms. Special stains (periodic acid–Schiff [PAS] and Gomori methenamine silver [GMS]) are sometimes necessary to demonstrate the organisms in cases with low numbers of fungal elements. If the organisms are not detectable on histopathology and fungal culture is negative, *Sporothrix*-specific immunofluorescence testing should be performed. A blood culture should be submitted if hematogenous dissemination is suspected.

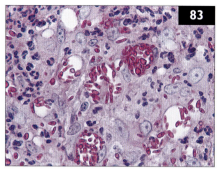

83 Case 83 is the same cat as in case 82. Histologically, diffuse pyogranulomatous dermatitis and intralesional yeast-like organisms were found (83) (PAS stain).
i. Which oral antifungal drug is recommended and how should the cat be treated?
ii. What are the public health risks and how can transmission be prevented?

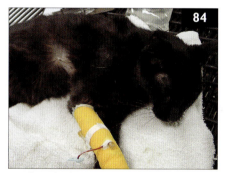

84 A 9-month-old intact female domestic shorthair cat was seen because of sudden onset of weakness, anorexia, and vomiting of 3 days' duration. On physical examination, the cat was subdued, severely dehydrated (84), and febrile (body temperature 41°C). The intestinal loops were thickened and rubbery, and mesenteric lymphadenopathy was apparent. Further questioning revealed that this cat had never been vaccinated. Because of clinical signs and the history, feline parvovirosis was suspected.
i. What are the clinical presentations of feline parvovirosis at different stages in a cat's life?
ii. How is feline parvovirosis diagnosed?
iii. How should this patient be treated?
iv. How is FPV transmitted?

83 i. The treatment of choice for cats is itraconazole (5–10 mg/kg PO sid) due to lower risk of side-effects compared to other commonly used oral antifungal drugs. It is imperative that the affected cat is treated for at least 1–2 months beyond complete clinical resolution. In cases with a lack of response to therapy or unacceptable side-effects, terbinafine (10–30 mg/kg PO sid) can be used as an alternative.

ii. Due to the high number of fungal organisms in the lesions of cats, sporotrichosis is considered an emerging zoonosis. Infection in people occurs most commonly through contact with the lesions and their exudates or feces from infected cats. Other possibilities are scratches or bites from infected cats or even contact with clinically healthy cats having had contact with an infected cat. Infected people often suffer from a cutaneolymphatic form characterized by pustular to nodular lesions on the face and extremities with secondary lesions ascending the lymphatic vessels. People handling cats with suspected sporotrichosis should wear disposable gloves, discard them after each use, and wash hands and forearms with disinfecting soap.

84 i. If a queen is vaccinated with a MLV FPV vaccine or is infected with FPV during pregnancy in early to mid-gestation, the kittens may be resorbed or aborted. In late gestation, the kittens may develop ophthalmic lesions, cerebral disease, or cerebellar hypoplasia. Within a litter, there may be varying degrees of neurologic effects. If a neonate becomes infected, it may similarly develop cerebellar hypoplasia and reversible lymphoid and bone marrow hypoplasia. Older kittens and unvaccinated adults develop lymphoid necrosis, intestinal necrosis, and bone marrow suppression. Exposed cats with adequate antibody titers against FPV (from maternal antibodies or vaccination) usually remain free of clinical signs.

ii. Feline parvovirosis is suspected based on the clinical signs in combination with typical changes in the complete blood count (i.e. severe panleucopenia). In cats that recover, leukopoiesis is commonly evidenced. The diagnosis is confirmed by demonstrating the parvovirus in fecal samples using in-house tests that detect parvovirus antigens, electron microscopy, or PCR.

iii. IV fluid therapy is critical for recovery. Antiemetics should be administered as needed in addition to IV broad-spectrum bacteriocidal antimicrobials to treat bacteremia associated with profound leukopenia and loss of the normal intestinal barrier. Plasma or whole blood transfusions may be required.

iv. FPV is excreted in the feces and is spread by fecal–oral or fomite transmission. It is highly contagious and resistant to inactivation.

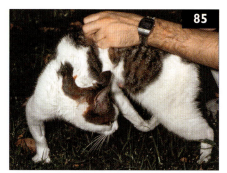

85 A 6-year-old spayed female domestic shorthair cat was seen because of localized tetanus with cervical musculature involvement (85). The cat was allowed to roam outside. The owner had first noted clinical signs, starting with stiffness, 5 days ago.
i. How should the cat be treated?
ii. What management options would have been indicated during the first 3 days of illness when the rigidity was developing?

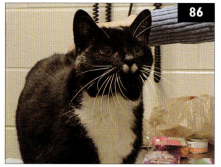

86 An 8-year-old castrated male domestic shorthair cat (86) was seen for a consultation. The cat came from a single-pet household in Germany. It was allowed to roam freely outside and to catch mice and birds. One day before presentation, the owner saw the cat eating a dead bird in the garden. The owner was very concerned because, 1 week before presentation, the district had been classified as a 'high risk district' for H5N1 avian influenza A virus. Some dead waterbirds found in a village about 5 km away were diagnosed with H5N1 avian influenza A. Subsequently, cat owners were told to keep their cats inside. In this case, however, the owner had not followed the advice.
i. Can cats become infected with avian influenza?
ii. How is the infection transmitted?

85 i. The following treatment is recommended: (1) The wound should be identified, cleansed, debrided of all necrotic tissue, and left open to inhibit anerobic growth of any remaining *Clostridium tetani*. (2) The cat should be treated with antibiotics (e.g. penicillin G and metronidazole). Ideally, antibiotics should be given intravenously (IV) or intramuscularly for the first few days. (3) If the spasms in the affected thoracic limb are of concern, centrally acting muscle relaxants such as diazepam (0.5 mg/kg PO q 8–12 h) can produce symptomatic relief. Methocarbamol can also be used for this purpose. (4) The prognosis in cases such as this is very good if only localized tetanus is present. Almost all animals make a complete recovery although it may require several months for normal limb function to return.
ii. In the initial stages of tetanus development, the possibility exists that localized tetanus may proceed to generalized tetanus, including involvement of the muscles innervated by the cranial nerves, as the toxin spreads throughout the neuraxis. It is therefore important to be much more aggressive when dealing with a developing case. In addition to antibiotics and extensive wound debridement, it would be prudent to administer tetanus antitoxin in the early stages of disease. As antitoxin is an equine immunoglobulin associated with a high rate of anaphylaxis, the toxin should first be tested intradermally (ID) or SC before the full amount is administered slowly IV.

86 i. Avian influenza is caused by infection with the H5N1 avian influenza A virus. Cats and other felids are naturally and experimentally susceptible to H5N1 avian influenza A virus infection. The highly pathogenic virus emerged in Hong Kong in 1997 and was transmitted from poultry to humans. After several years during which nothing was reported, the virus re-emerged in Asia, causing major lethal outbreaks in poultry and humans. Also, there were at least two outbreaks of fatal disease caused by the virus in tigers and leopards in Thailand. In Europe, two outbreaks occurred in cats in 2006 in Germany and Austria. Experimental infection with H5N1 avian influenza A virus of cats is possible; they develop a highly lethal disease.
ii. The transmission of H5N1 avian influenza A virus to mammals has occurred only sporadically. Cats can be directly infected by eating infected birds; cat infection is potentially highly dangerous because it may be associated with high morbidity and death rates as well as potential zoonotic risk. Also, in experimental studies, it has been shown that horizontal transmission between cats in contact can occur and depends on the amount of virus present. However, no cat–human transmission has been documented so far.

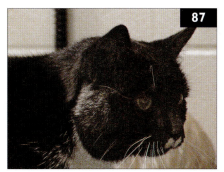

87 Case 87 is the same cat as case **86**. On physical examination, the cat appeared to be completely healthy (**87**).
i. What clinical signs do cats with H5N1 avian influenza A virus infection show?
ii. How can H5N1 avian influenza A virus infection be diagnosed in cats?

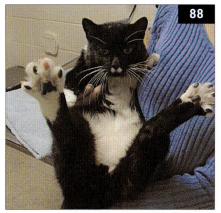

88 Case 88 is the same cat as cases **86** and **87**. The owner really loved the cat. It lived in very close contact with her, and usually slept in her bed, right next to her face (**88**).
i. Are cats a potential risk to humans?
ii. Can the disease be treated in cats?
iii. How can the infection be controlled in cats?

87 i. The incubation period is short: in experimentally infected cats, it was as short as 2 days, and in naturally infected large felids, it was reported to be 3 days. In infected cats, major clinical signs include fever, lethargy, protrusion of the nictitating membrane, conjunctivitis, nasal discharge, and labored breathing due to pneumonia. Generalized clotting disorders, icterus, and neurologic signs, including convulsions and ataxia, have also been reported. In severely affected cats, sudden death may occur as early as 2 days after the onset of clinical signs. Subclinical infections have also been observed.

ii. H5N1 avian influenza A virus infection should be suspected in the case of fever and acute respiratory symptoms in cats that have access to the outdoors in areas in which H5N1 avian influenza A virus infection has affected either poultry or aquatic wild birds. The clinical signs are not pathognomonic for the disease, and it may be difficult to differentiate from infections with FHV or FCV. Virologic diagnosis can be made on oropharyngeal, nasal, or rectal swabs, or fecal samples. At necropsy, affected organs, intestinal contents, and pleural fluid should be collected, and PCR should be performed. Viral antigens can also be identified by immunohistochemical techniques applied to sections of affected organs. Antibody detection can be performed (using hemagglutination inhibition tests), but these are likely to still be negative when clinical signs appear.

88 i. Potentially, cats could play a role in H5N1 avian influenza A virus transmission to other cats and humans. It is conceivable that the virus could adapt to cats, become less virulent, cause subclinical infections, and be propagated silently, with a potential risk of transmission to humans.

ii. At present, it is unknown whether antiviral chemotherapy is effective in cats.

iii. Control of H5N1 avian influenza A virus infection in cats and other susceptible pets (e.g. ferrets) can be achieved by avoiding contact with affected poultry or infected wild birds. Therefore, it is recommended to keep cats indoors in areas where avian cases of avian influenza have been reported. If a cat suspected of being infected is taken to the veterinary clinic, the veterinarian must take several measures to minimize the risk of transmission, including wearing gloves, mask, and goggles, isolating the cat, cleaning surfaces with a household detergent or a standard medical disinfectant, and reporting the case to public health officials. Recommendations for protection of the owner include minimizing contact with the cat and cleaning and disinfecting objects such as litter trays and bowls. At present, there are no vaccines against influenza for cats. In this case, oropharyngeal swabs were negative by PCR and the cat remained healthy. The owner promised to keep the cat strictly indoors for the time being.

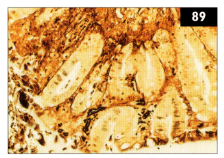

89 A 4-week-old intact male domestic shorthair kitten was seen because of a 2-day history of anorexia, diarrhea, and depression. All three littermates had died in the previous 5 days. On physical examination the kitten was approximately 10% dehydrated, mildly icteric, and minimally responsive. The kitten died before treatment could be instituted, and a necropsy was performed which revealed light-colored 1–2 mm scattered foci on the serosal and cut surfaces of the liver and on the ileocecocolic area of the intestine. Histopathologic sections of different organs, including intestines (89) (Warthin–Starry stain) were performed.
i. What is the most likely diagnosis?
ii. How is the diagnosis usually made?

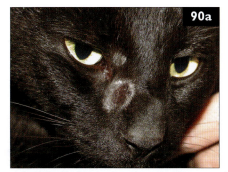

90 A 5-year-old spayed female domestic shorthair cat was seen because of suspected dermatophytosis. The cat showed pruritic circular alopecia in its face (90a).
i. What is dermatophytosis?
ii. What are the commonly used tests for the diagnostic evaluation of dermato-phytosis?
iii. What are the pitfalls of a Wood's lamp examination?

89 i. The most likely diagnosis is Tyzzer's disease (*Clostridium piliforme*). Disease outbreaks usually occur within litters of kittens, are infrequent, and the source of the infection is usually unknown. There is often a preceding history of immune deficiency or stress. The disease takes a rapid course, with death often occurring within 48 hours of the first clinical signs.
ii. As the disease progresses so rapidly, most diagnoses are made at necropsy, and little is known about premortem diagnosis or treatment options. The organism stains poorly with H&E but is readily visualized with special stains.

90 i. Dermatophytosis caused by *Microsporum canis* is a common disease in cats transmitted by contact with infected hairs, scales, and fungal elements. Clinical signs vary and may include circular alopecia, crusting, diffuse mild hypotrichosis, cutaneous hyperpigmentation, seborrhea, and generalized alopecia (**90b**). Pruritus is not usually present but can be severe at times. In rare cases, cutaneous nodules (dermatophytic pseudomycetoma) can be found.
ii. Due to this variation a diagnosis cannot be made by clinical signs alone. Wood's lamp examination, microscopic examinations of affected hairs, and fungal culture are indicated. Another test (e.g. skin biopsy) is sometimes necessary if the nodular form of dermatophytosis is suspected. However, in all other forms of the disease histopathology is considered less sensitive than fungal culture.
iii. The Wood's lamp should be used only as an initial screening test. Sensitivity of the Wood's lamp test is low because only 30–80% of *Microsporum canis* infections and virtually none of the other occasionally found dermatophytes (e.g. *Trichophyton mentagrophytes*, *Microsporum gypseum*) fluoresce. Typically a positive Wood's lamp test is characterized by bright green fluorescence along hair shafts (**90c**). False-positive reactions, caused by crusts (keratin), presence of *Pseudomonas* spp., lint, soap, petroleum or other topical drugs, do occur but usually are weak, vary in color, and affect structures other than hairs. Because of these pitfalls, suspicious hairs should always be cultured. The fluorescence is wavelength dependent and so it is recommended to warm up the Wood's lamp for about 5 minutes and to use lamps with power cords instead of battery-operated models.

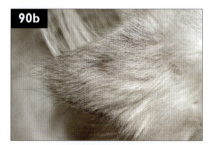

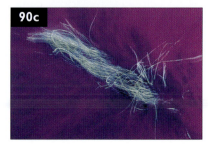

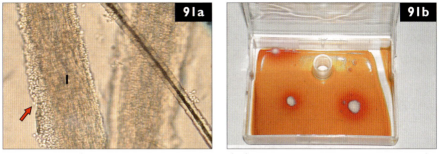

91 Case **91** is the same cat as case **90**. Wood's lamp examination was negative. The hair was examined in mineral oil under the microscope (**91a**, arrow, arthroconidia; 1, fungal hyphae). In the culture (dermatophyte transport medium [DTM]), a change of color was seen (**91b**). Cytologic examination of the culture was performed.
i. How effective is a microscopic examination of hairs?
ii. When is a dermatophyte culture considered positive for dermatophytosis?
iii. What is the diagnosis based on the cytologic examination of the culture?
iv. How should samples be collected from a cat suspected of dermatophyte infection but with no obvious skin lesions?

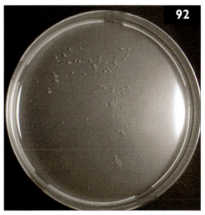

92 A 2-year-old spayed female domestic shorthair cat was seen because of a 2-day history of dyspnea, coughing, anorexia, and dehydration. It was an indoor/outdoor cat. Findings on physical examination included abnormal lung sounds and muffled cardiac sounds. Thoracic radiographs demonstrated a large amount of pleural effusion. Thoracocentesis revealed a purulent red-brown fluid containing small gray granules (**92**) with a high protein concentration (62 g/l) and a high leukocyte count (89 × 10^9/l), mainly consisting of degenerating neutrophils and macrophages.
i. What is this type of effusion called and what is the significance of the gray granules?
ii. What is the best method to confirm the diagnosis?
iii. What microbiological procedures should be performed?

91 i. If Wood's lamp-positive hairs are present, examination of such hairs is very helpful for making a preliminary diagnosis and to start therapy. Lack of fluorescing hairs, however, makes detection difficult and time-consuming. The typical microscopic findings are irregularly thickened hair shafts with loss of structure and fungal hyphae within the hairs. The surface of affected hairs is covered with small, clear, and round fungal spores called arthroconidia (**91a**).

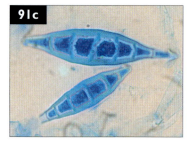

ii. Culture plates should be monitored daily for 21 days. A color change to red and the simultaneous development of a white-colored colony is suspicious for dermatophytes. However, to confirm the diagnosis a cytologic examination of the colony is necessary.

iii. Spindle-shaped, thick-walled macroconidia with six or more cells are seen (**91c**) (methylene blue stain). These features are diagnostic for *Microsporum canis*. Macroconidia can only be found on fungal cultures, but similar structures can occasionally be found on the skin surface representing saprophytic fungi.

iv. The best way to collect sample is the toothbrush (MacKenzie) method. With this method a sterile toothbrush is used to brush through the animal's coat collecting hair and keratin, which are subsequently inoculated onto the culture medium.

92 i. The fluid is considered an exudate. The presence of 'sulfur granules' suggests actinomycosis or nocardiosis. Both cause a suppurative to pyogranulomatous disease that may occur in a localized or disseminated form in cats (and dogs). Immunocompromised animals are at greater risk of infection. Clinical manifestations include abscesses in facial and cervical areas, abdominal abscesses, pyothorax, cutaneous granulomas, osteomyelitis or, rarely, disseminated disease. The route of infection is often by penetrating trauma.

ii. Diagnosis is made by cytology, histology, and culture of the organisms. Cytologic examination of exudates usually reveals pyogranulomatous inflammation and mixed bacterial populations. The presence of 'sulfur granules' is the best indicator of actinomycosis or nocardiosis. The granules consist of colonies of organisms; *Actinomyces* spp. appear individually or in dense mats (granules), as Gram-positive, nonacid-fast, branching, filamentous rods. *Nocardia* spp. aggregates contain Gram-positive, partially acid-fast, infrequently branching, filamentous rods with beading.

iii. Definitive diagnosis can be obtained by culturing the exudates for at least 4 weeks. It is not unusual to have negative cultures in some cases of actinomycosis or nocardiosis. The samples should be obtained anaerobically and an appropriate anaerobic transport culture medium should be used. In this case, *Nocardia* spp. were cultured.

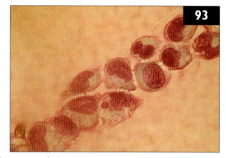

93 A 5-month-old intact male domestic shorthair kitten was seen with a 3-day history of shifting-leg lameness and reluctance to walk. On physical examination the kitten was approximately 8% dehydrated, febrile (body temperature 40.4°C), and had swollen appendicular joints that were painful to palpation. Joint fluid collected from a stifle was turbid and thin. Cytology of the fluid was evaluated (93) (Wrights–Giemsa stain).
i. What are the cytologic findings of the joint fluid?
ii. Which of the following is the most likely diagnosis?

A. Bacterial synovitis.
B. Calicivirus polyarthritis.
C. Rickettsial infection.

D. Immune-mediated polyarthritis.
E. Mycoplasmal polyarthritis.
F. Degenerative joint disease.

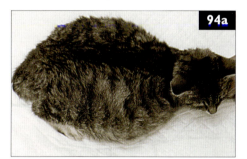

94 An 8-month-old intact female domestic shorthair cat was seen because of a sudden increase in abdominal size. The cat lived mainly indoors but was allowed to go outside in the garden. It was the only animal in the household. The cat had received its primary vaccination series. The owners had not noticed any sign yet of the cat being in estrus. It had not been spayed yet because, at the time of the surgical appointment, the cat had developed diarrhea, which later resolved without any treatment. Otherwise, the cat had been healthy. Massive abdominal distension was the only abnormality on physical examination (94a).
i. What are the rule-outs for abdominal distension?
ii. What are the diagnostic procedures that should be performed?
iii. What are the differentials for fluid in the abdominal cavity?
iv. If effusion is present, what would be the next diagnostic steps?

93 i. The joint fluid cytology shows a mononuclear infiltrate with a high-protein background. Bacterial, mycoplasmal, rickettsial, and immune-mediated arthritis produce neutrophilic inflammation with high cell counts. Degenerative joint disease does not generally affect multiple joints simultaneously in young animals, and cell counts are usually low with mixed inflammation.
ii. B, calicivirus polyarthritis. This is a classical presentation of 'feline limping kitten syndrome', in which kittens develop severe mononuclear polyarthritis and high fever following natural FCV infection or vaccination against FCV. Typical upper respiratory tract signs may or may not be present. Treatment is supportive care and analgesia, and full recovery without residual joint damage is expected to occur within 1 week. FCV was cultured from the stifle of this cat.

94 i. Potential rule-outs are effusion, pregnancy, pyometra, increase in organ size, or increased air content. The severe distension makes effusion and pregnancy the most likely causes in this cat.
ii. The next step is radiography and/or ultrasonography.
iii. The two major differentials for abdominal effusion are: (1) Leakage of normal body fluids into the abdominal cavity. This may include blood, bile, urine, or chyle. The fluid may be characterized by comparing laboratory values of the fluid to those of blood. (2) Presence of nonphysiologic fluids, including transudates, modified transudates, and exudates. Transudates, modified transudates, and exudates can be differentiated according to their cell content, protein content, and specific gravity. These are low in transudates, medium or mixed in modified transudates, and high in exudates.
iv. If there is effusion, a fluid sample should be evaluated; tests on effusions are much more useful, especially for diagnosing FIP, than tests on blood. Fluid collection can be performed either under ultrasonographic guidance (**94b**) or blindly. In the latter case, the cat should be suspended horizontally, holding the shoulders and the lumbar region. The abdominocentesis is then performed at the lowest point of the abdomen near the umbilicus about 1 cm to the side of the midline (**94c**). Abdominocentesis should be avoided if a generalized clotting disorder is suspected; a clotting profile should be conducted first.

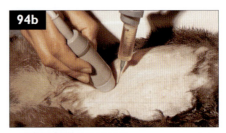

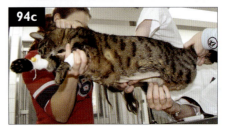

95 Case 95 is the same cat as case 94. A radiograph was taken and revealed effusion (95a). An abdominocentesis was performed. The effusion was yellow (95b) and of sticky consistency.

i. What is the prevalence of FIP among cats with abdominal effusion?
ii. What are the next diagnostic steps?
iii. How could FIP be confirmed in this case?

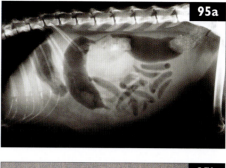

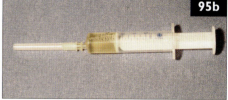

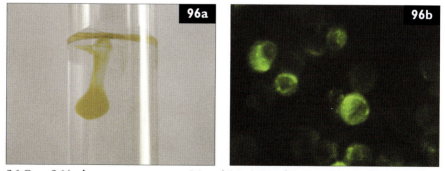

96 Case 96 is the same cat as cases 94 and 95. A Rivalta test (96a) and an immunofluorescence staining of FCoV antigen in macrophages of the effusion (96b) were performed.

i. What is the Rivalta test, and how should the result in this cat be interpreted?
ii. What is the interpretation of the FCoV immunofluorescence staining in this cat?

95 i. Only about half of cats with effusions have FIP. Thus, although effusions of clear yellow color and sticky consistency are often called 'typical', the presence of this type of fluid in body cavities is not diagnostic of FIP. In FIP, effusion is typically clear, straw colored, viscous, and may froth on shaking because of the high protein content. It may also clot when refrigerated. If the sample is bloody, purulent, foul smelling, or chylous, then FIP is less likely, although effusions in FIP can be very variable.

ii. Cell content, protein content, and specific gravity of the effusion should be examined. FIP effusions are usually classified as a modified transudate or exudate. The protein content is usually very high (>35 g/l), because of the high concentration of γ-globulins, whereas the leukocyte count is low (<5 × 10^9/l). Typically, LDH and α-amylase activities are high. Other diseases causing similar effusions include lymphoma, heart failure, cholangiohepatitis, pancreatitis, and bacterial peritonitis or pyothorax. FIP effusions typically show a pyogranulomatous character cytologically, whereas effusions associated with bacterial serositis or lymphoma often contain bacteria or malignant cells, respectively.

iii. The two tests that should be performed to confirm the diagnosis of FIP are the Rivalta test and detection of FCoV antigen in macrophages of the effusion using immunofluorescence staining.

96 i. The Rivalta test is very useful in cats to differentiate effusions due to FIP from effusions caused by other diseases. Three-quarters of a reagent tube are filled with distilled water, to which one drop of acetic acid is added, and mixed thoroughly. One drop of the effusion fluid is carefully layered onto the surface of this solution. If it disappears and the solution remains clear, the test is negative. If the drop retains its shape, stays attached to the surface or slowly floats down to the bottom, the test is positive. In cats, this test has a positive predictive value of 86% and a negative predictive value of 97%. There are some false-positive results in cats with bacterial peritonitis and lymphoma, but these can usually be differentiated cytologically. Overall, the Rivalta test is very practical and inexpensive, and does not require special laboratory equipment; it can easily be performed in private practice.

ii. Other methods to detect the virus itself include evaluation for the presence of FCoV antigen. Immunofluorescence staining of intracellular FCoV antigen in macrophages of the effusion is 100% accurate if this test is positive: it confirms the diagnosis of FIP. Unfortunately, there are some cases that stain negative although the cats have FIP; they can be explained by a low number of macrophages in the effusion of these cats.

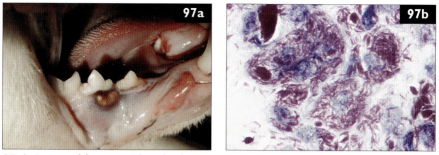

97 A 2-year-old castrated male domestic shorthair cat was seen because it was inappetant. The cat lived in the center of a big city. It had brought a dead rat home 4 weeks previously. On physical examination, the right mandibular lymph node was enlarged (2 × 1 × 1 cm) and several small nodules were observed in the gingival mucosa (**97a**). The cat had an elevated body temperature (39.9°C). A fine-needle aspirate was taken from the right mandibular lymph node (**97b**) (modified Ziehl–Neelsen stain).
i. What is the most likely diagnosis?
ii. How should the cat be treated?
iii. What are the potential complications of treatment?

98 A 7-year-old intact female domestic shorthair cat was seen because of neurologic complications of a bite wound and scratches on the head. It had been treated with long-acting penicillin, and the wound had been flushed with saline. The mental status of the cat deteriorated, however, and it experienced two short generalized seizures. On physical examination, there was some swelling over the left frontal and

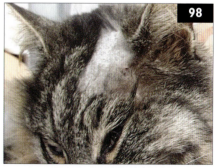

temporal bones and two small blood-encrusted scars (**98**). The body temperature was 37.9°C. The cat was stuporous and unable to stand. Postural reactions were absent in the right limbs and decreased in the left limbs. Menace responses were absent in both eyes. The pupils were small, but the pupillary light reflexes were present. Normal physiologic nystagmus was absent in both eyes.
i. What is the neuroanatomical localization of the lesion and the most likely differential diagnoses?
ii. What are possible risks associated with anesthesia?

97 i. In the aspirate, masses of acid-fast bacilli within the cytoplasm of macrophages in dense parallel accumulations are seen. The most likely diagnosis is feline leprosy, caused by *Mycobacterium lepraemurium*, the agent of murine leprosy, and other mycobacterial species, e.g. *M. visibile*. Cats infected with *M. lepraemurium* are thought to acquire infection from the bite of an infected rodent. They develop multiple cutaneous and/or subcutaneous nodules, most commonly on the head and forelimbs. Nodules are firm, haired or alopecic, and frequently ulcerate. Occasionally, as in this case, lesions occur in oral and/or nasal mucosa. Regional lymph node involvement is common. The disease is most prevalent in temperate climates and tends to mostly occur in young cats, especially during winter.

ii. The best approach to treatment is a combination of surgical resection of localized lesions combined with adjunctive antimicrobial therapy for 1–2 months beyond resolution of lesions. Disease recurrence is common after surgical excision alone. Combination antimicrobial therapy using clofazimine or rifampicin with clarithromycin and ciprofloxacin is usually curative. Spontaneous remission may occur occasionally, especially during the summer months.

iii. Potential complications of therapy include recurrence of lesions if therapy is not given for long enough, and drug toxicities. Clofazimine, an iminophenazine dye, and rifampicin, a macrocyclic antibiotic, may both cause reversible hepatotoxicity. Clarithromcyin, a new-generation macrolide, may cause generalized or pinnal erythema.

98 i. Abnormal mentation and seizures may be caused by intracranial disease, metabolic, or toxic causes. Here, cranial nerve deficits (absent menace response and oculocephalic reflexes), and UMN tetraparesis (worse on the right) indicate intracranial disease. Taken together, the neurologic tests suggest bilateral forebrain (seizures, absent menace response) and brainstem (UMN tetraparesis, no physiologic nystagmus) disease. This could be a diffuse or multifocal intracranial lesion or a large forebrain lesion with herniation and subsequent brainstem compression. Postural reaction deficits were more pronounced on the right limbs suggesting a lateralized lesion. Considering the history, both inflammation and trauma were considered.

ii. As there is probably increased intracranial pressure and imminent brain herniation, adequate ventilation and oxygenation must be ensured during general anesthesia for neuroimaging and surgery. The cat should be intubated and ventilated to avoid hypercapnia, and pCO_2 should be consistently monitored. Compression of the jugular veins should be strictly avoided because this may decrease venous return from the head and subsequently cause a fatal increase in intracranial pressure. MRI is more sensitive than CT for imaging pathological alterations within the neuroparenchyma such as abscesses, inflammation, hemorrhage and edema. However, its main disadvantage is the longer anesthetic time required, and the difficulty of patient monitoring during anesthesia.

99 Case **99** is the same cat as case **98**. Treatment was switched to cefotaxime and metronidazole, and fluid was supplied at maintenance rates. However, the cat died the following day.
i. What could have been done differently?
ii. What other drugs, besides antibiotics, should have been used?

100 A 10-year-old spayed female domestic shorthair cat was seen because of weight loss and decreased appetite of 1 month duration (**100**). The cat resided in an indoor/outdoor multi-cat household. About 2 months ago, the owner had noticed blood in the urine and straining. This was treated for 2 weeks, sucessfully for a while, with an antibiotic. Physical examination was incom-

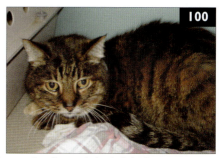

plete because the cat was aggressive. Radiographs showed the left kidney was very small, and there was gastric mineralization. On ultrasonography, the right kidney was hyperechoic and the right renal pelvis and proximal ureter were dilated. The left kidney was only 2 cm long and had no normal architecture. A complete blood count, biochemistry panel, and urinalysis were performed; the notable findings were:

Blood profile/biochemistry panel	Results
Band neutrophils	0.48×10^9/l
Creatinine	301 µmol/l
Urea	25 mmol/l
Urinalysis (cystocentesis)	
Color/appearance	yellow, hazy
Specific gravity	1.026
Blood	++++
RBC	Numerous
WBC	5–10 cells/hpf
Casts	0–1 coarse granular casts/hpf

i. What are the two major problems in this cat?
ii. How should each problem be assessed?

99 i. Treatment of bacterial encephalitis or brain abscess is usually started empirically with broad-spectrum antibiotics which cross the blood–brain barrier. Parenteral use of bactericidal drugs is preferred. Antibiotics effective against anerobic infections should be given for brain abscesses. The combination of cefotaxime and metronidazole fulfills these requirements. Alternatives would be chloramphenicol or sulfonamide–trimethoprim. Both are broad-spectrum and cross the blood–brain barrier. Clindamycin may express a potent postantibiotic effect through its accumulation within leukocytes beyond measurable CSF levels. Aminoglycosides and first-generation cephalosporins are not recommended for treatment of bacterial CNS infections.

ii. Brain edema and imminent brain herniation are usually addressed with immediate diuretic therapy with furosemide (1–2 mg/kg IV q 6–8 h) and mannitol (1–2 g/kg IV over 15–30 minutes). Anti-inflammatory dosages of dexamethasone (0.1–0.2 mg/kg) twice daily may be given during the first 2 days of treatment to decrease the proinflammatory action of cytokines. Higher dosages of dexamethasone may be required if there is sudden deterioration and brain herniation. Fluid therapy should be carefully planned. The goal is to maintain hydration, but overhydration should be strictly avoided because this may cause worsening of the neurologic status. Thus, rehydration may be best achieved using synthetic colloids (hetastarch) or hypertonic saline solutions. Because the cat had two generalized seizures, phenobarbital (1.5–2 mg/kg PO or IV q 12 h) should be started.

100 i. There are two major problems, (1) decreased appetite (combined with weight loss) and (2) azotemia.

ii. Problem 1 is decreased appetite and weight loss. One is probably the cause of the other. The pyuria on the urinalysis suggests inflammation in the urinary tract possibly causing the increased band neutrophil count. Problem 2, azotemia, explains the clinical findings. However, other possibilities should also be considered in this geriatric cat. Dental problems are possible; mild sedation is indicated to examine the mouth. Prerenal, renal, and postrenal causes of azotemia should be considered: (1) With a purely prerenal cause, the specific gravity should be >1.030. (2) With a postrenal cause, there should be evidence of rupture or obstruction of the urinary tract. (3) The urine specific gravity of 1.026, azotemia, and abnormal kidneys strongly suggest that this azotemia is renal in origin.

The next question with renal azotemia is whether the renal failure is acute or chronic. In this case, the finding of gastric mineralization and the small left kidney along with the vagueness and duration of clinical signs support chronic renal failure. The dilated renal pelvis and proximal ureter in the right kidney could be due to bacterial infection (pyelonephritis) or to partial proximal ureteral obstruction. The urinalysis suggests that there is hemorrhage and inflammation in the urinary tract. This could be from the upper or lower urinary tract.

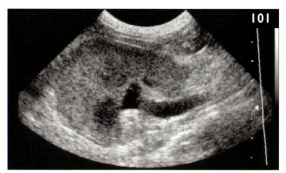

101 Case 101 is the same cat as case 100. Pyelonephritis is suspected in this cat. Partial ureteral obstruction is another diagnostic possibility. The right renal pelvis and the proximal right ureter were dilated on ultrasonography (101).
i. What further diagnostic testing should be done?
ii. What treatment should be provided at this point?

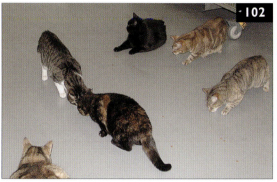

102 A 10-year-old intact female domestic shorthair cat was seen because of dermatophytosis. The cat lived in a cattery with a group of 23 cats. Eight of these cats showed skin lesions suspicious for dermatophytosis (102).
i. What are the three main goals for getting this problem under control?
ii. How should affected cats be identified and how should they be treated?
iii. Does the environment need to be decontaminated?
iv. How should the response to therapy be monitored and what should be recommended regarding prevention?
v. What are the concerns regarding public health?

101 i. Further diagnostics should include a urine culture. An excretory urogram could be performed, but is often unrewarding in azotemic animals due to reduced excretion of contrast. The only test that could determine whether infection is from the upper tract is direct sampling of urine from the renal pelvis under ultrasound guidance for cytology and culture, which would be ideal here. Contrast agent could also be injected into the renal pelvis to evaluate for ureteral obstruction.
ii. Symptomatic therapy for the moderate azotemia should include IV administration of a balanced electrolyte solution. The amount should equal 3% dehydration plus maintenance. An alkalinizing balanced electrolyte solution such as lactated Ringer's (administered at 18 ml/h IV for 24 hours) would be appropriate. Additional fluids should be administered if excessive losses occur. The level of azotemia (and hyperphosphatemia, if present) should be reassessed in 24 hours. If the azotemia improves, but the appetite continues to be reduced, the cat should be sedated for a thorough oral examination. Medical management for chronic renal failure should be instituted. Antibiotic therapy should be delayed until the urine culture is returned, as no bacteria were seen on urinalysis, and the cat was treated with antibiotics in the recent past.

102 i. There should be separation of carriers from noncarriers, aggressive treatment of infected animals, and measures to prevent reinfection.
ii. Samples for fungal culturing should be obtained from all of the cats. If the strain is Wood's lamp positive, this is useful for finding infected cats and to monitor response to therapy. Cats with obvious or suspected infection must be quarantined, as must the whole cattery. Topical therapy should be started in all cats immediately. Once fungal culure results are available, all cats with positive results should also be treated with systemic antifungal therapy. The most commonly used drugs are itraconazole (5–10 mg/kg PO sid) for 3 weeks or alternating weeks, and microsize griseofulvin.
iii. Decontamination of the environment is very important. The most effective and most commonly used disinfectants are household bleach (2%) and enilconazole.
iv. The response to therapy should be monitored by fungal culture. Samples should be collected every 2 weeks until two consecutive tests are negative. Cats not responding to treatment should be removed. Eradication in a cattery can take up to 6 months. To prevent introduction of dermatophytosis, all cats entering a cattery should have a fungal culture performed, followed by an antifungal dip (e.g. lime sulfur), and then quarantined until two consecutive fungal cultures are negative.
v. Dermatophytosis is a zoonotic disease and a risk factor for children, cancer patients, and people with other immunocompromising diseases.

103 A 7-month-old intact male domestic shorthair cat was seen because of progressive small bowel diarrhea of 1 week's duration. It had been found 3 weeks previously, and had tested negative for FeLV and FIV at that time. It had received one dose of pyrantel pamoate and two vaccinations against FPV, FHV, FCV, and FeLV and one vaccination against rabies. It was fed a

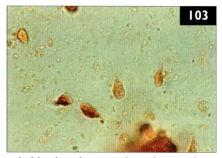

commercially available kitten chow and resided both indoors and outdoors. There were two other adult cats in the household, both healthy. On physical examination, the kitten was depressed, very thin, and had a poor hair coat. Dehydration was estimated at 6%. Vital signs were within normal limits. Abdominal palpation was unremarkable. A direct fecal smear (103) and fecal flotation were performed.
i. What is the diagnosis?
ii. What treatment is recommended?
iii. Is environmental management indicated?
iv. If so, what recommendations should be made to the owner?

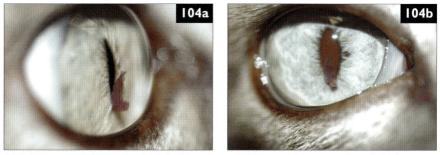

104 A 7-year old castrated male Siamese cat was seen because of a pinkish mass-like object in the right eye (104a) and a subtle color change of the iris from a blue to a yellow-blue (104b). The owner reported that the eye had been cloudy, red, and painful on a previous occasion. The cat lived in a single-cat household, and had outdoor access. The owner also had two dogs. The cat was current on all vaccinations, and a recent test for FIV antibodies and FCoV antibodies was negative. An ophthalmic examination was performed; significant results were: PLR (direct and indirect) L + R + (very brisk); IOP L 19 mmHg R 10 mmHg.
i. What is the ocular diagnosis for the right eye based on the initial findings and ophthalmoscopic examination?
ii. How can the color change of the right iris be explained?

103 i. The diagnosis is giardiasis. The fecal smear shows *Giardia* spp. trophozoites.
ii. Fenbendazole is effective in dogs, but has not been critically evaluated in cats. Furazolidine is also effective in cats, but may cause vomiting and diarrhea. Metronidazole may be used, but metronidazole-resistant strains of *Giardia* spp. exist. The efficacy of the *Giardia* vaccine is controversial. Vaccination should only be used therapeutically in cats with giardiasis in addition to drug therapy. Fluid therapy is indicated in this case, and a bland, highly digestible diet should be used until the diarrhea resolves.
iii. *Giardia* spp. cysts persist in the environment for several months if conditions are wet and cold. Environmental decontamination is essential for the successful treatment of giardiasis.
iv. Environmental management should consist of the following: (1) Treat all animals with drug therapy as above and move out of the environment to a holding area. (2) Disinfect the environment using a quaternary ammonium compound. (3) Bathe all animals with a general pet shampoo. (4) Then bathe animals again with a quaternary ammonium compound (particularly the perineum); ammonium compounds should not be left on longer than 3–5 min and should be rinsed thoroughly. (5) Return animals to the disinfected environment after bathing.

104 i. The pinkish mass within the anterior chamber is a blood-tinted fibrin clot, attached to the iris. The anterior chamber is otherwise clear. The IOP in the right eye is much lower than in the left eye. Low IOP (hypotony) and fibrin accumulation in the anterior chamber are signs of anterior uveitis. This cat probably had a more severe bout of inflammation previously (as the owner reported a cloudy, red, and painful eye). Uveitis refers to inflammation of parts of, or the entire uveal tract. The clinical signs vary, but aqueous flare, fibrin accumulation, hyphema, and iris color change are most consistently observed in cats. Clinical signs are caused by breakdown of the blood–aqueous barrier located in the ciliary body. In this cat, the ophthalmoscopic examination also revealed multiple inactive scars in the tapetum indicative of a previous bout of chorioretinitis. Similar to the blood–aqueous barrier, the blood–retina barrier normally prevents leakage of fluid from the choroid into the subretinal space. This barrier is compromised during inflammatory processes, usually an infection.
ii. Color change of the iris is a commonly observed clinical sign in uveitis and is especially dramatic in light-colored (blue) irides. A blue iris may become reddish-brown, and a brown iris may become darker or depigmented. The iris color change in acute inflammation is reversible but may become permanent in chronically inflamed eyes.

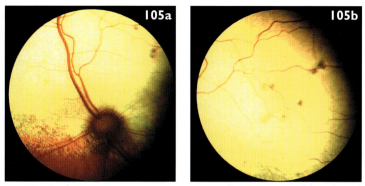

105 Case 105 is the same cat as case 104. Both eyes were dilated with 0.5% tropicamide for further examination. The ophthalmoscopic examination revealed multiple inactive chorioretinal scars (105a) in the tapetum of the right eye (105b).
i. What are possible etiologies, given the ophthalmologic findings?
ii. What diagnostic tests should be performed?
iii. How should the cat be treated?

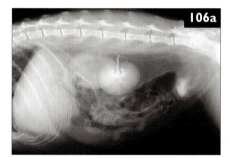

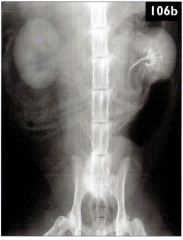

106 A 14-year-old spayed female domestic shorthair cat was seen because of inappetence and vomiting for 3 days. On physical examination, the cat had a high body temperature (39.7°C), and the right kidney appeared painful. An abdominal ultrasound examination showed a normal left kidney, right pyelectasia, and right hydroureter. An IV urogram was performed. Lateral (106a) and ventrodorsal (106b) radiographs were taken 3 minutes postcontrast injection.
i. What are the findings in the IV urogram?
ii. What are the differential diagnoses?
iii. How should this case be further investigated?

105 i. In cats, the most common causes of uveitis are infectious diseases. Among those toxoplasmosis, systemic mycoses, FIP, bartonellosis, mycobacteriosis, and infections with FHV, FeLV, and FIV are differentials.

ii. In all cats with uveitis, a thorough physical examination and a complete blood count, biochemistry panel, and urinalysis are recommended; these were all normal here. Infectious disease testing is also indicated. The results in this cat were all negative for the following: FeLV antigen and PCR, FCoV antibody, FIV antibody, systemic fungal infection serology (cryptococcosis antigen, histoplasmosis antibody, blastomycosis antibody, coccidiomycosis antibody), *Bartonella henselae* antibody. However, tests for *Toxoplasma gondii* IgM and IgG antibody titers measured twice, 1 week apart, showed a rising IgM antibody concentration. This shows active *T. gondii* infection, and that this is the cause of the ocular lesions. A thoracic radiograph was normal. *T. gondii* is frequently the cause of anterior uveitis in cats, although usually there are no concurrent systemic signs.

iii. Treatment in this cat consisted of topical prednisolone acetate and flurbiprofen. The cat also received oral clindamycin (10–12.5 mg/kg bid) for 4 weeks. The fibrin in the anterior chamber disappeared, and the IOP in the right eye normalized. It is prudent to regularly recheck cats with previously diagnosed *T. gondii* uveitis, as the formation of immune complexes of *T. gondii* and other antigen-driven immune processes may perpetuate a chronic low-grade uveitis.

106 i. The right kidney is larger than the left. There is opacification of the renal parenchyma bilaterally. There is a normal pyelogram and ureterogram on the left side with no evidence of contrast accumulation or excretion in the right kidney. Together with ultrasound, these findings are consistent with right hydronephrosis and hydroureter secondary to a right ureteral obstruction.

ii. The differential diagnoses are ureteral obstruction with inflammatory debris or blood secondary to pyelonephritis or ureteritis, ureteral urolith, or ureteral tumor.

iii. A percutaneous, ultrasound-guided, right renal pelvic aspirate and cystocentesis should be performed for urinalysis and culture. If infection is present, the cat may be treated conservatively with antimicrobial therapy. The intravenous urogram could be repeated in 24–48 hours to determine right ureteral patency. Other options include CT urography or exploratory laparotomy and cannulation of the right ureter, plus insertion of a nephrostomy tube for temporary urine diversion if patency cannot be established immediately. In this case, the renal pelvis aspirate contained masses of inflammatory cells and bacteria. A pure growth of *Escherichia coli* was found in the culture. Concurrent ureteritis was suspected. An IV urogram repeated 24 hours after starting antibiotic therapy showed no relief of ureteral obstruction. The cat was given a single dose of prednisolone sodium succinate (4 mg/kg IV). A third IV urogram 48 hours later demonstrated ureteral patency. The cat made a complete recovery.

107 A 7-year-old castrated male domestic shorthair cat (107) was seen because of pyrexia (body temperature 40.7°C) and lameness of its right hind leg. The cat was allowed to roam freely outside and commonly spent the nights outside. It was routinely vaccinated and wormed. Besides the high body temperature, physical examination was unremarkable, and orthopedic examination was not able to localize the hind leg

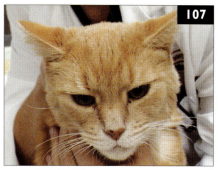

problem. Joints of both hind legs were unremarkable. The owner was concerned about Lyme disease as the owner's father had had Lyme disease and the cat was from an endemic area and sometimes had ticks.
i. Can cats develop Lyme disease?
ii. Can *Borrelia* spp.-infected cats be a risk to humans?

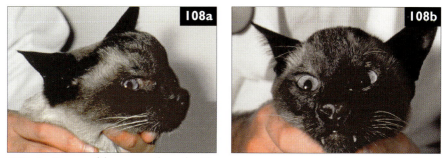

108 A 7-year-old neutered male Siamese cat was seen because of a large subcutaneous swelling on its forehead over the frontal sinus region. This subcutaneous swelling had been present for several weeks and was growing in size. Upon close questioning, the owner indicated that the cat had also had some inspiratory stertor and nasal discharge over the same period. The cat was otherwise well. Physical examination was unremarkable, apart from mild mandibular lymph node enlargement, swelling of the bridge of the nose (108a), and some crusty nasal discharge (108b).
i. What are the differential diagnoses?
ii. What are the prognoses for these possibilities?
iii. What is the most cost-effective way of making a diagnosis?

107 i. Lyme borreliosis is overdiagnosed in veterinary medicine because it has become a 'trendy' disease. The presence of antibodies to *Borrelia* spp. signifies exposure to a spirochete but does not prove that current clinical illness is caused by the organism. In endemic areas, many animals, including cats, in the population have antibodies without ever developing clinical signs. Cats can be antibody-positive, and experimental infection has been produced, but naturally acquired disease has rarely been documented. This cat developed an abscess over the pelvis on the right side that most likely resulted from a bite of another cat. The abscess was drained, and the cat was treated with antibiotics. Fever and lameness resolved after 2 days.

ii. There is no evidence that human infections have occurred after contact with infected cats (or dogs). Infected cats could only, potentially, pose a risk to humans by introducing unfed tick stages into a household. Direct horizontal spread from cats to people is unlikely. Although Lyme disease is classified as a zoonosis, cats, dogs, and people are incidental hosts for a sylvan cycle that exists in nature. Lyme borreliosis in humans is usually associated with outdoor activities that result in exposure to tick vectors.

108 i. The cat has nasal cavity disease, which would appear to be progressive and invasive. The disease process had penetrated through the bones overlying the nasal cavity to involve the subcutaneous tissues over the nasal bridge. The differential diagnoses include: (1) Nasal cavity neoplasia, including adenocarcinoma, squamous cell carcinoma, chondrosarcoma, osteosarcoma, and lymphoma. (2) Mycotic rhinitis, including cryptococcosis, aspergillosis, *Neosartorya* infections, and phaeohyphomycosis. (3) A foreign body within the nasal cavity (included for completeness, but unlikely to be associated with such invasive disease).

ii. The prognosis for the fungal diseases and foreign bodies is favorable, although treatment can be expensive and protracted. The prognosis for intranasal neoplasia is generally poor, although many cases of nasal lymphoma respond favorably to multi-agent chemotherapy and/or radiotherapy.

iii. Although there are various ways of investigating this case, the most cost-effective way would be to obtain a sample of the abnormal tissue causing the subcutaneous swelling over the bridge of the nose. This tissue is likely to be representative of whatever disease process is occurring in the nasal cavity, and is easier to access. Two or three fine-needle aspirates should be obtained for cytologic evaluation. It is usually possible to do this under light sedation. If cytology is inconclusive, a larger portion of tissue should be obtained using a core biopsy device or *via* surgical excision of the abnormal tissues under general anesthesia.

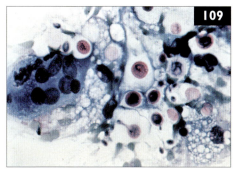

109 Case 109 is the same cat as case 108. The fine-needle aspirate showed large numbers of capsulated yeasts demonstrating narrow-necked budding (109).
i. What is the organism in the fine-needle aspirate?
ii. Are nasal swabs (taken for cytologic examination and culture) likely to be useful in such a case?
iii. Are radiographs of the nasal cavity likely to provide useful diagnostic or prognostic information?
iv. How should the cat be treated?

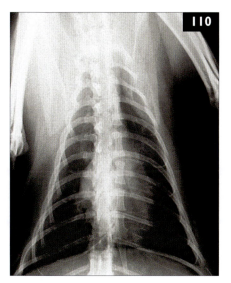

110 A 3-year-old castrated male domestic shorthair cat was seen in Italy because of an intermittent cough. Thoracic radiographs showed a diffuse pulmonary interstitial pattern and enlargement of the right caudal lobar and peripheral pulmonary arteries. The cardiac silhouette was unremarkable (110).
i. What is the most likely differential diagnosis for the radiographic findings in this cat?
ii. What clinical signs are expected in this disease in cats?
iii. What further tests should be performed?

109 i. This morphology is strongly suggestive of cryptococcosis. In this case, a fine-needle aspirate was plated onto Sabouraud's dextrose agar and bird-seed agar, and *Cryptococcus neoformans* was isolated subsequently.

ii. Nasal swabs are useful for diagnosing cryptococcosis. In this case, only small numbers of yeasts were present in smears made from nasal swabs. However, as a general rule, material in the subcutaneous tissues over the nasal bridge (if present) is likely to provide a better sample than nasal exudate.

iii. Usually, nasal radiographs and CT provide little or no extra useful information concerning diagnosis or treatment in these cases. CT demonstrates the extent of bony invasion and destruction, and whether the cribriform plate has been breached.

iv. Treatment should consist of a combination of surgery and antifungal drug therapy. As much fungus-impregnated tissue as possible should be removed surgically prior to commencing drug therapy. Accordingly, the subcutaneous mass over the nasal bridge was debulked in this case, and the cat was treated with fluconazole for 6 months. To reduce drug costs, ketoconazole was administered for an additional 8 months. There was a very satisfactory response to treatment. It is important to monitor therapy using sequential antigen tests. Ideally, the cat should be treated for at least 2 months after the antigen titer declines to zero. In this cat, disease recurred after 14 months of 'maintenance' ketoconazole therapy.

110 i. There is enlargement of the lobar and peripheral pulmonary arteries with loss of tapering and occasional tortuosity and truncation. These findings are characteristic of heartworm disease (dirofilariasis) in cats. However, radiographic features suggestive of feline heartworm disease are found in only 53% of cases.

ii. Cats with feline heartworm infection may be asymptomatic or have chronic respiratory signs such as intermittent cough, increased respiratory effort, and dyspnea. Rarely, a systolic heart murmur may be present in cats with heartworms in the right atrium and ventricle. In acute exacerbation, signs may include salivation, tachycardia, tachypnea, hemoptysis, vomiting, and diarrhea. Serous and chylous pleural effusion, ataxia, blindness, vestibular signs, and syncope may occur but are uncommon. Some cats can die suddenly. Acute death has been widely reported in asymptomatic cats infected with heartworms, due to an acute pulmonary arterial infarction, specifically acute pulmonary thromboembolism, after spontaneous death of adult heartworms. The bronchial signs are frequently a consequence of immature adult heartworms which never become fully adult, and cause heartworm-associated respiratory disease (HARD). The clinical signs of this syndrome are nonspecific and, on initial presentation, it may be impossible to distinguish them from asthma, pulmonary parasitism, diffuse bacterial pneumonia, or fungal disease.

iii. Antibody and antigen tests for *Dirofilaria immitis*, echocardiography, and BAL (to rule out other diseases) are useful additional tests.

111 Case 111 is the same cat as case 110. A complete blood count revealed mild eosinophilia (1.9 × 10⁹/l). BAL fluid cytology showed a large number of eosinophils. The antibody test for *Dirofilaria immitis* was positive and the antigen test was negative. The owner decided to euthanize the cat due to financial concerns, and a necropsy was performed. Histology of lung tissue confirmed inflammation and presence of *D. immitis* (111).

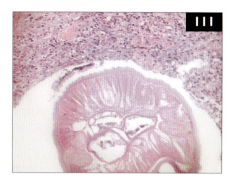

i. What laboratory changes are expected in a cat with heartworm disease?
ii. How can the results of the heartworm tests be interpreted?

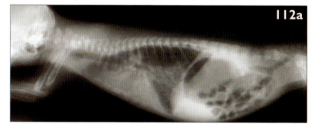

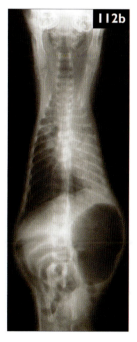

112 A litter of four 9-day-old domestic shorthair kittens was seen because of fading kitten syndrome. The kittens were active and had nursed vigorously at birth. A fifth kitten died the previous day after 24 hours of progressive dyspnea, cessation of suckling, crying, and progressive abdominal distention. At presentation, one of the four surviving kittens was hypothermic (body temperature 34.8°C), dyspneic, and exhibited abdominal distention and weakness. It had a body weight of only 125 g (expected weight for this age: 150–200 g). The three other kittens appeared healthy. Lateral (112a) and ventrodorsal (112b) radiographs were taken of the dyspneic kitten.

i. What is the most likely diagnosis?
ii. What are the appropriate diagnostic procedures?

111 i. In cases of feline heartworm disease, hematologic and biochemical abnormalities are nonspecific. A mild nonregenerative anemia is present in about one-third of infected cats. Some cats have hyperproteinemia due to hyperglobulinemia, sometimes combined with hypoalbuminemia, and some cats may develop glomerulonephritis-associated changes (e.g. proteinuria). BAL cytology may reveal a large number of eosinophils 4–7 months postinfection. However, eosinophilia is a nonspecific and inconsistent finding and its absence does not exclude heartworm disease.
ii. Interpretation of antibody and antigen test results is complicated. The negative antigen test indicates that there are no adult female worms present. The antibody test is usually positive in earlier stages of infection during the larval phase with parasites of either sex. However, positive antibody tests only document exposure and not current infection or clinical illness. Results of both tests should be considered carefully.

112 i. The most likely diagnosis is fading kitten syndrome due to bacterial sepsis and bronchial pneumonia. The ventrodorsal radiograph demonstrates extensive consolidation of the lungs, aerophagia, and gastrointestinal ileus. This is especially obvious when compared to lateral (**112c**) and ventrodorsal (**112d**) radiographs of one of the healthy littermates. Fading kitten syndrome is the most common cause of death in kittens 1–6 weeks of age. The route of infection may be *via* the respiratory tract, gastrointestinal tract, umbilicus, or by undetermined routes, and infection frequently spreads to multiple organs. Frequently, low total IgG concentrations are documented. Neonatal sepsis typically affects entire litters.

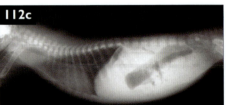

ii. The collection of large volumes of blood for extensive testing is impossible, but a small amount of blood can be collected by jugular venipuncture for selected tests or a blood smear evaluation. Whole body radiographs can be performed. The queen should receive a thorough evaluation: physical examination, complete blood count, serum biochemical panel, urinalysis, and tests for FeLV and FIV. If she is to be used in a breeding program, vaginal cultures for *Streptococcus canis* should be performed. Milk should be expressed from each gland and evaluated for evidence of mastitis visually and by cytology if necessary. A necropsy including microbiological cultures should be performed on the dead kitten and any others that die.

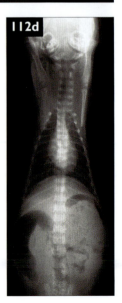

113 Case **113** is from the same litter as case **112**. The sick kitten was euthanized due to its current suffering and the poor prognosis for recovery once clinical signs of neonatal sepsis develop. Both dead kittens were submitted for necropsy, which revealed omphalophlebitis (umbilical infection) and abscessation of multiple organs. *Escherichia coli* and *Streptococcus canis* were isolated from the tissues. This kitten stopped nursing so a nasogastric tube was placed for nutritional support and hydration (**113**).
i. How should the surviving kittens be treated?
ii. What is their prognosis?

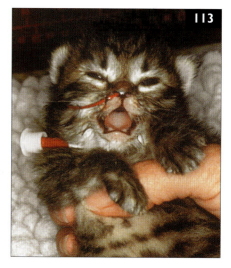

114 A 6-year-old neutered male domestic shorthair cat was seen because of blepharospasm and epiphora of the right eye. The ophthalmic examination revealed a corneal opacity in the nasal quadrant of the eye and mild bilateral conjunctivitis. After one drop of corneal anesthetic (topical proparacaine), a white tubular worm, about 10 mm long, was observed moving on the outer surface of the cornea (**114**).
i. What is the diagnosis?
ii. What are the clinical signs of this infection?
iii. What diagnostic procedures should be performed?
iv. What treatment is indicated?

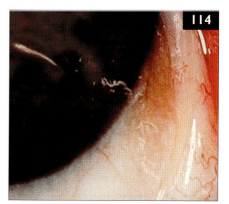

113 i. Treatment of litters experiencing neonatal sepsis should be aggressive and involve the entire litter, regardless of each kitten's current status. Once signs of sepsis develop, survival is unlikely. Broad-spectrum parenteral antibiotics should be administered SC to all kittens for a minimum of 10 days. Critically ill neonates should receive antibiotics by IV or IO routes. Oral absorption of antibiotics in neonates is not reliable. In general, kittens should receive antibiotic dosages normally used in adults unless specific information is available to guide dose alterations. Fluid balance and nutrition can be maintained by nasogastric intubation if required. If necessary, a needle can be inserted into the humerus or femur for vascular access. Passive immunity can be provided to supply antibacterial antibodies. A total of 15 ml of serum collected from a healthy cat and administered in divided doses (5 ml SC q 12 h) at birth results in normal serum IgG content in colostrum-deprived kittens.

ii. The prognosis for kittens already exhibiting signs of sepsis is poor. In contrast, aggressive therapeutic intervention for kittens not yet showing signs of disease is likely to be successful in a majority of cases. Kittens surviving to weaning are expected to grow normally without lasting consequences of early infection. All three kittens in this litter survived with aggressive supportive care.

114 i. The cat was infested with an eyeworm. The most common eyeworms are *Thelazia callipaeda* and *T. californiensis*. They are spiruroid roundworms which are approximately 10–19 mm long, live on the conjunctiva of the eye, and produce irritation and lacrimation.

ii. Clinical signs are due to L3 and L4 larvae and adult worms in the conjunctival sac; they can irritate the conjunctiva and damage the cornea, resulting in conjunctivitis, mild corneal opacification, corneal scarring, and profuse lacrimation. Other parasitic diseases that may be associated with similar ocular signs are ocular acanthamebosis and onchocercosis.

iii. The primary diagnostic procedure is thorough ophthalmic examination of the eye after topical anesthetic administration (proparacaine drops). In cats, one to two *Thelazia* spp. adult worms may be found under the nictitating membrane and eyelids, while in dogs five or more worms may be observed.

iv. Usually no treatment other than mechanical removal is required. Administration of topical or systemic ivermectin, levamisole, or moxidectin prior to parasite removal may be useful. In dogs, moxidectin as ocular drops or SC may be useful in preventing disease.

115 An approximately 16-week-old intact female domestic shorthair kitten was seen because of a nonhealing wound on the ventral cervical area (115). The kitten had been found as a stray 2 weeks previously and appeared to be otherwise healthy. Physical examination was normal with the exception of a 2-mm hole in the skin over the trachea. There was minimal inflammation and drainage.
i. What is the most likely diagnosis?
ii. What is the appropriate treatment?
iii. What is the prognosis?

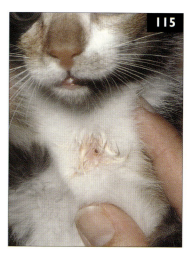

116 A 9-year-old castrated male Siamese cat was seen because of collapsing episodes that were becoming more frequent; the cat had experienced five episodes during the preceding 2 weeks. The cat reportedly became stiff immediately before collapsing, and these episodes were preceded by periods of labored respiration. The cat had experienced two similar episodes 6 months earlier. Each episode lasted only a few seconds. The cat was also reported to have vomited two to three times a week over the preceding few months. Vomiting was unrelated to eating. On physical examination, a mild systolic murmur was auscultated over the cat's sternum. Its heart rate was regular (150 bpm) and breath sounds were harsh. Lateral and ventrodorsal (116a) thoracic radiographs were taken.
i. What is the interpretation of the thoracic radiographs?
ii. What differential diagnoses could account for the historical, physical, and radiographic findings?
iii. How should the cat be treated?

115 i. The physical findings are classic for *Cuterebra* myiasis.

ii. Treatment involves enlarging the cutaneous breathing hole and gently extracting the living parasite larva with forceps. Care is taken to avoid damaging the parasite *in situ* as hypersensitivity reactions can result. Antibiotics are indicated postsurgery if there is evidence of inflammation.

iii. The prognosis for a full recovery following removal of the parasite is excellent. In most cases, only a single parasite is present. Occasionally, larvae are found in the respiratory tract or other tissues where more significant clinical signs can develop. The kitten should be started on a preventive health program, including core vaccinations appropriate to its environment, internal and external parasite control, and testing for FeLV and FIV. The first vaccine was administered at the time of *Cuterebra* removal. The wound had healed completely by the following visit 3 weeks later.

116 i. The thoracic radiographs demonstrate enlargement of the left and right caudal lobar pulmonary arteries and a generalized bronchointerstitial pattern. Also, the left caudal lobar pulmonary artery appears truncated.

ii. The presence of significant cardiopulmonary disease suggests the events described by the owners were syncopal episodes. The findings of enlargement and pruning of pulmonary lobar arteries, in concert with a bronchointerstitial pattern and a history of vomiting strongly suggest heartworm disease (dirofilariasis). On echocardiography, one or more heartworms (*Dirofilaria immitis*) are seen in the right ventricular outflow tract straddling the pulmonary valve. A portion of a heartworm is viewed as hyperechoic parallel linear bands (**116b**), and three pairs of hyperechoic dots are evident (**116c**), representing a heartworm in transverse section. Vomiting is also probably caused by heartworm disease, although why this happens is unclear.

iii. The cat was treated with prednisolone and exercise restriction. This reduces cardiopulmonary manifestations of hypersensitivity to filarial antigens. In this case, no further episodes of syncope occurred. The dose of prednisolone was maintained for 3 months, and then gradually tapered. Adulticide therapy using thiacetarsamide or melarsomine is generally considered too dangerous as primary therapy for feline heartworm infection. Surgical retrieval of heartworms represents another option, especially if the worms are visualized echocardiographically in an accessible position, such as the right atrium or vena cava.

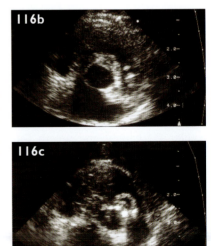

117 An 8-year-old neutered female domestic shorthair cat was seen because of lethargy and anorexia for 3 days (117). The cat lived strictly indoors, there were no other pets in the household, and the cat did not have contact with any other animals. It had been vaccinated twice, at the ages of 6 and 10 weeks. On physical examination, the cat was very lethargic and slightly dehydrated.

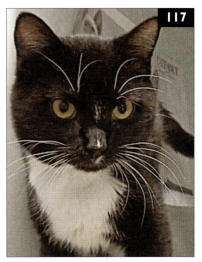

Blood profile	Results
Platelets	89×10^9/l
WBC	0.4×10^9/l
Mature neutrophils	0.02×10^9/l
Band neutrophils	0
Lymphocytes	0.25×10^9/l
Monocytes	0.01×10^9/l

i. What is the pathophysiology of the leukopenia?
ii. Can a strictly indoor-living cat develop feline panleukopenia?
iii. Can a cat be infected from a dog?
iv. Can a dog be infected from a cat?
v. Does the vaccine protect cats from infection with a canine parvovirus?

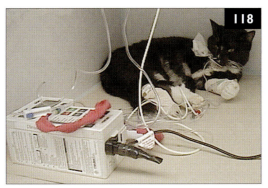

118 Case 118 is the same cat as case 117. The cat had panleukopenia and was treated intensively (118).
i. What symptomatic treatment is appropriate in a cat with panleukopenia?
ii. Which antibiotics should be used?

117 i. The leukopenia in this cat is caused by both a neutropenia and a lympho-penia. The neutropenia is severe and is due to insufficient production or destruction of neutrophilic precursors, as no band neutrophils are present, thus there is no sign of regeneration.

ii. Parvoviruses are extremely stable and can remain infectious for more than a year. Thus, the owner could have carried the parvovirus into the house and exposed the cat.

iii. The canine parvoviruses now circulating in the dog populations worldwide (CPV-2a, CPV-2b, CPV-2c) are able to infect cats and to cause disease that is indistinguishable from parvovirosis caused by FPV. In this case, the cat was infected with a canine parvovirus that the owner had brought into the apartment by stepping in dog feces that was contaminated with virus. The leucopenia in this cat can be explained by replication of the parvovirus in neutrophils and lymphocytes. The thrombocytopenia is likely caused by DIC commonly present in panleukopenia.

iv. Dogs cannot be infected with FPV. However, as a cat with panleukopenia may be infected with a canine parvovirus, the cat with panleukopenia should be considered to be a potential risk to dogs.

v. The feline vaccine also protects cats from infection with canine parvoviruses. However, this cat was last vaccinated against FPV at 10 weeks of age. Maternal antibodies were probably still present at this age and interfered with effective immunization. It is recommended that the final kitten vaccine should not be given until at least 16 weeks of age.

118 i. A cat with panleukopenia should be kept in isolation and receive intensive care. (1) IV fluid therapy is the most important treatment. This should be continued for as long as vomiting and diarrhea persist. (2) Metabolic acidosis and hypokalemia are common and should be corrected through additions to the IV fluids. (3) Oral intake of water and food should only be restricted if vomiting persists and should be restarted as early as possible. (4) If persistent vomiting occurs, antiemetics should be considered. (5) If hypoproteinemia develops, plasma or whole blood may be required. Serum albumin concentration should be maintained at 20 g/l or higher. If edema is present it should be corrected by a plasma transfusion or synthetic colloids, such as hetastarch. In severe cases, partial or total parenteral nutrition (TPN) may be required. (6) Cats with panleukopenia can, rarely, develop thiamine deficiency. Vitamin supplements can be given to prevent this.

ii. The gut barrier is often destroyed, so intestinal bacteria may easily enter the blood stream. Sepsis may ensue in these immunocompromised patients. Thus, antibiotics should be administered parenterally, ideally IV. As bacteria derive from the gut, an antibiotic with good efficacy against Gram-negative and anerobic bacteria is recommended (e.g. third-generation cephalosporins).

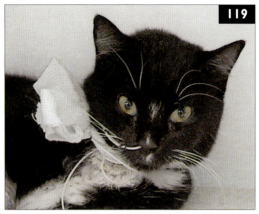

119 Case 119 is the same cat as cases 117 and 118. Although treated intensively, the cat was not improving and additional treatment options were considered (119).
i. Are drugs available that increase the neutrophil count?
ii. Is interferon treatment useful?
iii. Is administration of specific antibodies useful?

120 A 15-year-old spayed female domestic shorthair cat was seen at the emergency service. The cat was an indoor only cat, and was obese (BCS 4.5/5). The cat ate everything it could find and was usually alone in the apartment throughout the day. The owner was concerned because when she came home from work 2 hours before presentation she found that the cat had eaten the contents of a can of beef that the owner had opened the day before but then discarded because the can had ballooned and was 1 year over the expiry date. On the radiographs (120), food was seen in the cat's stomach.
i. What disease can occur if spoiled canned food is ingested?
ii. Can cats get the disease?

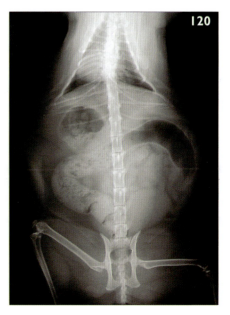

119 i. Filgastrim (G-CSF) has been used in both cats and dogs with parvovirus-associated neutropenia, but is ineffective. Also, in cats it may lead to an increase in FPV replication; thus, it is not recommended.

ii. Feline interferon-ω has recently been licensed in many European countries and in Japan for the treatment of cats (and dogs). There are no clear data on the treatment of cats with panleukopenia; however, there is proven efficacy of feline interferon-ω in dogs with parvovirosis. Thus, a beneficial effect might be expected in cats as well.

iii. Specific antibodies can be used both as prevention and for treatment of parvovirus infection. Commercial products containing highly concentrated immunoglobulins (multi-valent hyperimmune immunoglobulin preparations) are available in some European countries for cats as heterologous preparations produced in horses, containing a combination of antibodies against FPV, FHV, and FCV. The protective effect of these antibodies lasts about 3 weeks. If used prophylactically, active immunization (vaccination) is not recommended for 3 weeks. Repeated treatment (with an interval of more than 1 week) is not recommended in cats because it may cause anaphylactic reactions due to antibody production against equine antigens in the preparation. In addition to these commercial products, SC administration of immune serum or hyperimmune serum is possible. Serum can be stored for 1 year if frozen promptly after collection.

120 i. The owner is concerned about botulism. *Clostridium botulinum* is a Gram-positive, spore-forming, saprophytic, anerobic rod that is distributed in soil worldwide. Botulism is caused by a neurotoxin produced by the organism that causes neuromuscular paralysis. In order to cause disease, either the organism or its spores must contaminate a food source. Most cases in animals are caused by ingestion of the preformed toxin in food. Naturally-occurring botulism in dogs has been mainly attributed to eating carrion or raw meat.

ii. Although botulism has been experimentally produced in cats, no natural cases of botulism have been reported. A cat that ate contaminated yogurt did not become ill even though two humans eating the same yogurt did. Produced under experimental conditions, the disease in cats is similar to that occurring in dogs because botulinal neurotoxins cause similar signs in all species. Although there are no reports of natural disease in cats, cats can be the source of outbreaks in cattle. Recently, 427 Holstein cattle died from botulism; they had been fed a rotten bale of oat hay containing a dead cat, and botulinum toxin C was identified. The cat in this report was kept in hospital for observation. No clinical signs occurred and the cat remained healthy. However, it was admitted for a weight-reduction program.

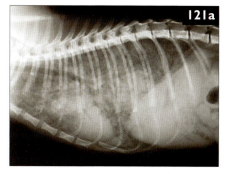

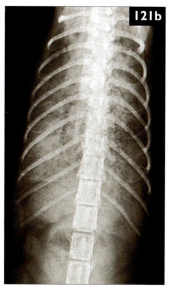

121 A 1-year-old intact male domestic shorthair cat was seen because of a 2-day history of nonproductive cough and dyspnea. The cat was an indoors/outdoor cat regularly vaccinated against FCV and dewormed with pyrantel at 3 months of age. Lateral (121a) and ventrodorsal (121b) radiographs were taken.

i. What are the radiographic findings?
ii. What are the differential diagnoses for the problems of this cat?
iii. What is the diagnostic plan?

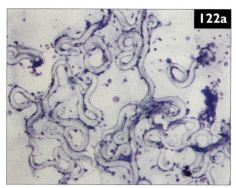

122 Case 122 is the same cat as case 121. BAL was obtained from the cat (122a).
i. What diagnosis do the BAL findings support?
ii. What are the typical findings in this disease?
iii. What secondary problems may complicate the disease?
iv. What treatment should be performed?

121 i. The radiographs show a diffuse mixed interstitial and alveolar pattern with air bronchograms that could be caused by various lung tissue diseases, including bronchopneumonia, severe edema, or hemorrhage.
ii. Differential diagnoses include systemic diseases such as fungal infection (e.g. cryptococcosis, histoplasmosis), FIP, toxoplasmosis, neoplasia (e.g. lymphoma, tumor metastases), lungworm infection, hemorrhage, and edema.
iii. A complete blood count, biochemistry panel, urinalysis, fecal examinations, FIV and FeLV test, *Toxoplasma gondii* IgG and IgM antibody titers, and BAL should be performed. Tests for FeLV antigen, FIV antibodies, *T. gondii* antibodies, and fecal sedimentation as well as flotation were negative in this cat. The complete blood count showed mild eosinophilia (1.7×10^9/l). All other laboratory values were within normal limits.

122 i. A large number of lungworm larvae, identified as *Aelurostrongylus abstrusus*, were found. Lungworms are an important cause of chronic coughing in endemic areas and should be considered in the diagnostic workup of coughing cats. *A. abstrusus* infects the cat when it eats the intermediate hosts (e.g. snails, slugs) or paratenic hosts (e.g. rodents, amphibians, birds). After the eggs hatch, the larvae migrate into the bronchi and trachea where they are coughed up and swallowed.
ii. Eosinophilia ($>1.0 \times 10^9$/l) is commonly present. L1 larvae (370 μm in length) may be found in fecal samples using the Baermann flotation test. Microscopic diagnosis is not useful before the fifth to sixth week of infestation and after the fourth month after infestation. In BAL, a high number of eosinophils may be observed, and L1 larvae (**122b**) may be present in the exudates.
iii. Secondary bacterial or fungal infections can occur as a result of chronic lesions in the lung, complicating the clinical course. Therefore, the tracheal or bronchial wash fluid should also be submitted to bacterial culture.
iv. Fenbendazole is the drug of choice to treat lungworm infection. Corticosteroids can be used for acute clinical manifestations due to the antigen release from larval death in the lung. Inhalant albuterol and corticosteroids may also be useful.

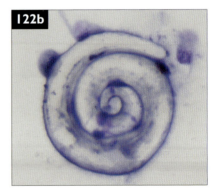
122b

123 A 3-year-old spayed female domestic shorthair cat was seen because of a mild head tilt to the left, intermittent falling on turns and when shaking the head, and anisocoria. It was an indoor-only cat. Neurologic examination showed Horner's syndrome of the left eye characterized by miosis, ptosis, and enophthalmos (123) but was otherwise unremarkable.

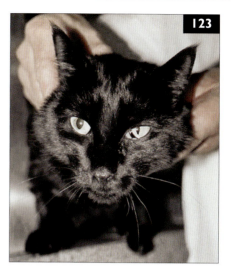

i. What is the neuroanatomical location of the lesion?
ii. What are the likely differential diagnoses?
iii. What diagnostic procedures are warranted?

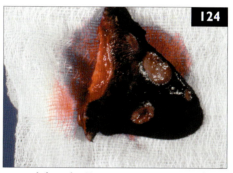

124 A 10-year-old spayed female Siamese cat was seen because of an abnormal looking ear. According to the owners, the problem had started as a single lesion of the tip of the left pinna. This lesion grew progressively larger and later became ulcerated. Three additional lesions of varying size but similar appearance developed subsequently in different parts of the pinna (124). The cat did not appear to be distressed by the lesions, and remained systemically well. Apart from the affected ear, the general physical and dermatologic examinations were unremarkable. The other ear was completely normal.

i. What disease processes could cause ear lesions such as this affecting only one ear?
ii. How can a definitive diagnosis be made?

123 i. Head tilt to the left and falling are evidence of vestibular disease. This may be of peripheral or central origin. There was no evidence on neurologic examination to suggest central vestibular disease; thus, the anatomic diagnosis is peripheral vestibular disease. Horner's syndrome is frequently seen with middle ear disease in cats.

ii. Rhinitis and pharyngitis can lead to otitis media *via* the Eustachian tube. Other causes of middle/inner ear disease are nasopharyngeal polyps (invading up the Eustachian tube), previous ear cleansing, and neoplasia.

iii. Further diagnostic evaluation should include imaging of the tympanic cavity. This is best achieved with CT or MRI. If advanced neuroimaging techniques are not available, radiography could be performed. In this cat, otoscopic examination revealed otitis externa and a defect in the tympanic membrane. Thus, the clinical signs were probably caused by middle and inner ear disease. Cytology revealed bacterial infection and the cat was treated systemically with antibiotics. After 2 weeks, the cat was re-examined and the clinical signs had improved markedly.

124 i. The differential diagnoses for multiple fleshy, ulcerated cutaneous lesions of an extremity would include: (1) Neoplasia, including squamous cell carcinoma and lymphoma. (2) Granulomatous or pyogranulomatous inflammation, including cryptococcosis, sporotrichosis, nocardiosis, mycobacteriosis, and foreign body reaction. (3) Allergic or traumatic cutaneous disease (unlikely).

ii. In this cat, the lesions are suggestive of an infectious or neoplastic etiology. However, considering the neoplastic conditions that commonly affect the skin and subcutis of the pinna, squamous cell carcinoma would seem unlikely as the cat had darkly pigmented ears, only one ear was affected, and the lesions looked fleshy rather than ulcerated. Multiple enlarging lesions are suggestive of an infection. To make a definitive diagnosis, it is necessary to take a biopsy for cytology, microbiology, histopathology, and in some instances PCR assay. Alternatively, a less invasive first approach would be to obtain a fine-needle aspirate from a representative lesion for cytologic assessment. It would be dangerous to remove the ear without at least obtaining material for histopathology, in case the disease process spreads to other sites later, or recurs at the site of surgical excision. In this case, Wrights–Giemsa-stained impression smears from the cut surface of an excised lesion demonstrated pyogranulomatous inflammation (neutrophils and macrophages) and pleomorphic yeast-like organisms, including oval and cigar-shaped forms. This is strongly suggestive of sporotrichosis.

125 Case 125 is the same cat as case 124. *Sporothrix schenkii* was isolated on Sabouraud's dextrose agar, and stained positive with PAS on histologic sections (125).
i. How did the cat become infected?
ii. What treatment options are available?
iii. Is amputation of the ear always indicated?

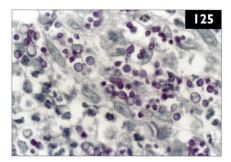

126 A 5-year-old castrated male domestic shorthair cat was seen because of hematuria and frequent urination (126a) for the past few days. It was kept completely indoors and was regularly vaccinated. When it was 2 years old, it had had several bouts of urethral obstruction and a perineal urethrostomy had been performed. The cat was fed an acidifying commercial dry diet. On abdominal palpation, the bladder felt small and the wall felt thickened. Abdominal radiographs showed radio-opaque uroliths in the urinary bladder (126b).

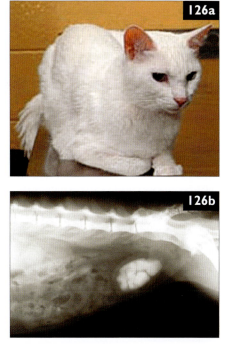

Urinalysis	Results
pH	8.0
Blood	++
Protein	++++
RBC	Numerous
WBC	10–50 cells/hpf
Casts	0
Squamous cells, fat globules	Many

Because of the presence of uroliths, pyuria, and hematuria, urine was obtained by cystocentesis for culture. This detected *Proteus* spp.
i. What are the cat's problems?
ii. What are the differential diagnoses?

125 i. Sporotrichosis results from inoculation of an organism, normally present in the soil, into cutaneous and subcutaneous tissues of the patient; infection may spread by local extension and *via* the lymphatics. The infection can potentially affect humans.

ii. The disease should be treated with surgery, followed by treatment with itraconazole or fluconazole (antifungal drugs). In this cat, surgical excision of the pinna was performed. The cat should be subsequently treated with itraconazole or fluconazole for a minimum of 4 weeks following surgery, to minimize the possibility of disease recurrence.

iii. In this case, if the owners had not been prepared to have the ear removed, it would have been acceptable to treat the cat initially with itraconazole. Itraconazole has good activity against *S. schenkii*, and it is likely that a long course of therapy could eliminate infection. However, if a prompt clinical improvement is not evident soon after starting therapy, amputation of the ear would be strongly recommended. Unfortunately, this is less acceptable in cases which involve more important structures, such as limbs. However, itraconazole can be hepatotoxic, but keto-conazole is much less likely to be effective for sporotrichosis and is not recommended. Also, the cat's owners should be made aware of the zoonotic potential of *S. schenkii*.

126 i. The presenting problems are hematuria and dysuria. The urinalysis indicates microscopic hematuria with pyuria. The urine pH is alkaline. Radio-opaque uroliths are evident on radiographs. The urine culture confirms a UTI. Both the cystoliths and a lower tract UTI can cause the presenting clinical signs.

ii. The cat had UTI due to *Proteus* spp. *Proteus* spp. may be urea splitters, leading to urine alkalinization. UTI is unusual in young cats, especially males. However, perineal urethrostomy predisposes to UTI. Persistently alkaline urine associated with infection with urea splitting organisms occurs despite feeding an acidifying diet. The alkaline urine causes the magnesium, ammonium, and phosphate normally present in feline urine to be less soluble, leading to magnesium ammonium phosphate (struvite) uroliths. Struvite uroliths associated with infection and markedly alkaline urine are typically large and radio-opaque as in this case. Struvite uroliths that form in sterile, acidic urine in cats are usually small and less radio-opaque, as less struvite precipitates when the urine is acidic. Calcium oxalate uroliths are also radio-opaque. They more commonly form in acidic urine. However, the only way to confirm that these cystoliths are struvite is to perform a mineral analysis of the uroliths.

127 Case **127** is the same cat as case **126**. A UTI with *Proteus* spp. was diagnosed in this cat.
i. What is an appropriate further diagnostic plan?
ii. What therapy is indicated?

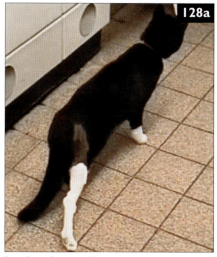
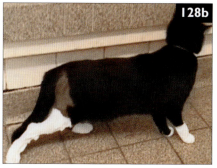

128 A 6-year-old spayed female domestic shorthair cat was referred because of a 5-day history of right pelvic limb paresis. It was allowed to go outside and was current on vaccinations (FPV, FHV, FCV, rabies). The cat was bright, alert, and responsive and moved freely around the room with the affected limb extended caudally (**128a**). The right popliteal lymph node was enlarged. The right pelvic limb had very little voluntary movement. Abnormal findings on neurologic examination were restricted to this limb, and included absent postural reactions, normal patellar and cranial tibial reflexes, and no withdrawal reflex. However, intermittently, the toes were placed correctly without knuckling (**128b**). Painful stimuli applied to the toes provoked an attempt at withdrawal, yet the limb remained extended. Radiographic examination was normal.
i. What is the neuroanatomic localization of the lesion?
ii. Which infectious agent could be a likely cause?
iii. How should this be treated?

127 i. This should include a complete blood count to see if there is a systemic inflammatory response. This is unusual with purely lower urinary tract disease. If an inflammatory leukogram is present, pyelonephritis should be considered. A biochemical panel should be performed to assess further the cat's renal function. Evaluation of calcium for hypercalcemia is important. The presence of hypercalcemia with radio-opaque uroliths makes calcium oxalate uroliths more likely.

ii. The UTI requires antibiotic therapy. The drug of choice is ampicillin or amoxicillin, since the organism is sensitive to these, they are reasonable in price, reach high concentrations in the urine, and have few side-effects. There are two therapeutic options for the uroliths. One is to remove the uroliths by cystotomy; another is to assume the uroliths are struvite and attempt medical dissolution with a calculolytic diet and antibiotics. Struvite uroliths treated in this way can dissolve in 1–3 months, but this approach requires that the cat remains on antibiotics for 4 weeks beyond radiographic dissolution of the uroliths. Radiographs should be re-evaluated at monthly intervals. Regardless of which approach is chosen, the cat should be monitored for resolution and recurrence of UTI to prevent urolith re-formation. This should be done initially by re-evaluating a urine culture and urinalysis at 1 and 2 months post-therapy and 3–6 months thereafter.

128 i. There was severe monoparesis of the right pelvic limb and no limb flexion, even when pressure was applied in this cat (**128c**). Postural reactions were decreased, and the patellar reflex was normal. Thus, there was upper motor neuron monoparesis due to an ipsilateral T3–L3 spinal cord lesion, or severe muscle stiffness (from contracture or fibrosis).

ii. The most likely infectious cause is localized tetanus, caused by *Clostridium tetani*. This was suspected in this case because close inspection disclosed a small wound on the paw. A characteristic feature of tetanus is the simultaneous contraction of flexor and extensor muscles, although, clinically, there is extension of the limb, due to the greater strength of the extensor muscles. In dogs and cats, both localized and generalized tetanus may occur. Localized tetanus starts with stiffness of one muscle or one limb closest to the wound; it may progress to generalized tetanus, or the disease may be self-limiting.

iii. In the present case, treatment consisted of surgical wound debridement, antitoxin, and metronidazole. Tetanus antitoxin is equine in origin, so there is a high risk of anaphylaxis on injection. To avoid this, a small test dose should be given subcutaneously 30 minutes earlier. Alternative antibiotics include penicillin G, clindamycin, and tetracycline. The cat recovered completely within 4 weeks.

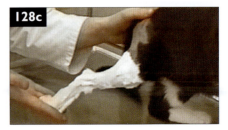

128c

129 A 5-year-old spayed female domestic shorthair cat was seen in Italy because of small disseminated cutaneous nodules and a crusting dermatitis around the eyes, head, neck, and pinnae (**129**). Physical examination revealed a thin cat (BCS 2/5), with peripheral generalized lymphadenopathy.

Blood profile/biochemistry panel	Results
Hematocrit – mild nonregenerative anemia	0.28 l/l
Reticulocytes	0
Hyperproteinemia	97 g/l
Hypoalbuminemia	22 g/l
Hyperglobulinemia	75 g/l
Polyclonal gammopathy – by serum electrophoresis	
Urea	52 mmol/l
Creatine	245 µmol/l
Urinalysis	
Specific gravity	1.027

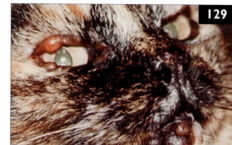

i. What are the most likely differential diagnoses in this cat?
ii. What are the next diagnostic steps?

130 Case **130** is the same cat as case **129**. FeLV antigen, FIV antibody, and *Toxoplasma gondii* antibody tests were negative. Fine-needle aspirates of skin nodules, eyelid lesions, and lymph nodes were obtained (**130**).
i. What are the main cytologic findings in this lymph node aspirate?
ii. What other tests could be performed?
iii. How common is this disease in cats and what is the prognosis for the cat?

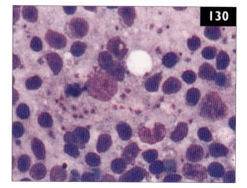

129 i. In adult cats, the most common form of anemia is a nonregenerative anemia due to inflammatory diseases. Elevated total protein is most commonly associated with chronic antigenic stimulation and resulting hypergammaglobulinemia. Taking all this into consideration, the differential diagnoses include chronic inflammatory diseases with dermatologic involvement such as parasitic infection (e.g. leishmaniasis), fungal infection (e.g. cryptococcosis), algal infection (e.g. prototheosis), neoplasia (e.g. mast cell tumor, lymphoma), systemic bacterial infections (e.g. mycobacteriosis), or autoimmune diseases.

ii. Further diagnostic tests include antinuclear antibody (ANA) tests (which are less reliable in cats than in dogs), fine-needle aspirates of cutaneous lesions and lymph nodes, and FeLV and FIV tests. The nonregenerative anemia associated with hyperproteinemia and polyclonal gammopathy is suggestive of systemic infection or inflammation. A bone marrow examination should be performed. Skin biopsies should be obtained if the skin aspirates are nondiagnostic. Ultrasonic imaging of the abdomen would help to characterize the azotemia.

130 i. Cytology shows small lymphocytes, some lymphoblasts, and macrophages with protozoon amastigotes containing a round basophilic nucleus resembling *Leishmania* spp.

ii. If cytology was nondiagnostic, further testing for *Leishmania* spp. antibodies, PCR of blood and bone marrow samples, and histopathology of cutaneous, eyelid, and lymph node lesions could be perfomed.

iii. Leishmaniasis is rare in the cat, but there has been a recent increase in cases of feline leishmaniasis in Spain, France, and Italy. In a series of eight cats with leishmaniasis in Italy in 2004, the main laboratory findings included mild nonregenerative anemia, thrombocytopenia, and hyperproteinemia with polyclonal hypergammaglobulinemia. Three of the cats had mild chronic renal insufficiency at the time of diagnosis. Severe pancytopenia with erythrocyte autoagglutination was found in a 4-year-old DSH cat in Portugal. Relative lymphocytosis and an increase in ALT were statistically associated with seroreactivity to *L. infantum*. Most of the cats examined, with or without treatment for leishmaniasis, developed severe renal failure with marked proteinuria. Thus, the prognosis in feline leishmaniasis is poor.

131 Case **131** is the same cat as cases **129** and **130**. A *Leishmania* spp. antibody titer was 1:64 (moderate titer). Bone marrow aspirates and PCR were positive for leishmaniasis. Using molecular techniques, the etiological agent was identified as *L. infantum*. Histopathology of cutaneous lesions showed a cellular infiltrate of aggregates of macrophages, lym-

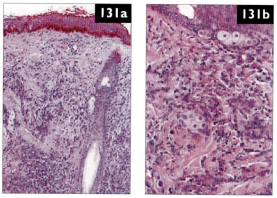

phocytes, and a few plasma cells. Numerous protozoan amastigotes were observed in macrophages in subcutaneous tissue at low (**131a**) and high (**131b**) magnification.
i. What are the main clinical features of the disease?
ii. What are the therapeutic options?

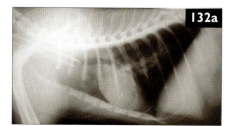

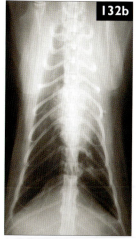

132 A 7-month-old spayed female Australian Mist cat was seen because of a 3-month history of paroxysmal coughing. During these episodes, the cat was seen to crouch, extend its neck, cough repeatedly, and then breathe rapidly and shallowly. The cat had been vaccinated against FPV, FHV, FCV, and FeLV and had no other history of being ill in the past. Abnormal physical findings included increased body temperature (39.3°C), mild mandibular lymphadenomegaly, and wheezes on thoracic auscultation. Gentle tracheal palpation induced severe coughing accompanied by respiratory distress. Complete blood count and biochemical profile were unremarkable. Lateral (**132a**) and ventrodorsal (**132b**) thoracic radiographs were taken.
i. What is the interpretation of the radiographs?
ii. What diagnostic procedure should be performed next?
iii. How should the cat be treated?

131 i. The main dermatologic signs include crusty ulcers, symmetric alopecia, and small nodules on the lips, nose, eyelids, and edge of the ear pinna. Lymphadenopathy is also reported and weight loss may occur secondary to glomerulonephritis.

ii. Treatment of feline leishmaniasis has not been established due to the small number of reported cases. Allopurinol seems to be a good therapeutic option. One cat with a nonhealing, ulcerated nodule on a hind leg, however, was unresponsive to treatment with allopurinol for 3 months, but was treated successfully by removing the lesion surgically. Some cats have been treated with meglumine antimoniate combined with ketoconazole with some success.

132 i. Thoracic radiographs demonstrate a diffuse bronchoalveolar pattern and consolidation of the left cranial lung lobe.

ii. Unguided or guided BAL or deep bronchial washing should be done next. In this case, unguided BAL was performed under general anesthesia. Stained smears of the lavage specimen showed large numbers of neutrophils and smaller numbers of eosinophils, alveolar macrophages, and lymphocytes. However, no bacteria were seen, so a portion of the BAL specimen was inoculated onto sheep blood agar plates and incubated aerobically and anaerobically (at 37°C). After 96 hours, a heavy growth of a monomorphic colony type was observed. Gram-staining of colonial material showed no bacteria. The colony morphology and lack of visible bacterial cells on Gram-staining were considered typical of a *Mycoplasma* spp. and no further identification procedures were undertaken. *Mycoplasma* spp.-induced bronchopneumonia was diagnosed on the basis of these findings.

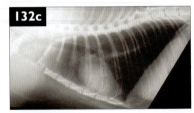

iii. The cat was discharged with doxycycline for 6 weeks. The cough resolved during the first week of therapy and the cat's general condition also improved. Radiographs taken after 6 weeks of treatment showed significant improvement on the lateral (**132c**) and ventrodorsal (**132d**) views. Antimicrobial susceptibility tests for *Mycoplasma* spp. have not been standardized and are not widely available. *Mycoplasma* spp. are reported to be sensitive to macrolides, azalides, lincosamides, tetracyclines, chloramphenicol, and fluoroquinolones.

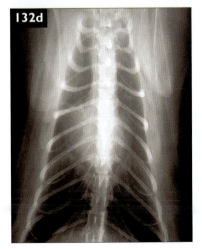

133 A 13-week-old intact female domestic shorthair kitten was seen because of an acute onset of severe respiratory distress. It had been coughing harshly for 2 weeks previously. It lived in a rural area. The kitten had been treated by a veterinarian at 6 weeks of age when it had been seen because of diarrhea, vomiting, and a high body temperature (40.1°C) with amoxicillin/ clavulanate PO for 7 days, and the clinical signs resolved. On physical examination, the kitten had a high respiratory rate (100 bpm) and a high body temperature (39.7°C). Thoracic radiographs were taken (133).

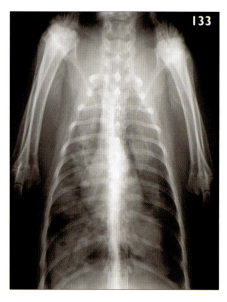

i. What are the abnormalities in the radiographs?
ii. How should the kitten's problems be investigated further?
iii. What are the differential diagnoses?

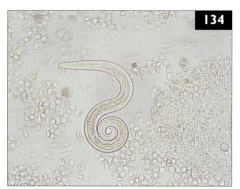

134 Case 134 is the same cat as case 133. A pure growth of *Salmonella enterica* serovar *typhimurium* was isolated from the bronchial wash fluid, and a structure was found in the bronchial wash fluid (134) (wet preparation).
i. What is this structure?
ii. What is the likely pathogenesis of concurrent salmonellosis and infection with the parasite in this kitten?

133 i. There is a bilateral pneumothorax, worse on the left, with an alveolar pattern in all lung lobes, patchy radiolucent foci, and irregular lung margins.
ii. The pneumothorax should be drained and an indwelling thoracostomy tube should be placed if the pneumothorax persists. A BAL should be performed with cytologic examination and culture of the sample collected. Alternatively, cytology of an ultrasound-guided fine-needle aspirate from consolidated lung could be performed. The kitten should be tested for FeLV and FIV. Feces should be collected for fecal sedimentation and flotation for the detection of lungworm larvae or ova, respectively.
iii. The differential diagnoses include parasitic (e.g. *Aelurostrongylus abstrusus*, *Eucoleus aerophila*, *Paragonimus kellicotti*), bacterial (e.g. *Escherichia coli*, *Pasteurella multocida*, *Klebsiella pneumoniae*, *Bordetella bronchiseptica*, *Mycoplasma* spp., *Streptococcus* spp.), protozoal (e.g. *Toxoplasma gondii*), or mycotic (e.g. *Cryptococcus* spp., *Histoplasma capsulatum*, *Blastomyces dermatitidis*) pneumonia.

134 i. The structure shown is the L1 larvae of *Aelurostrongylus abstrusus*. Larvae possess a characteristic S-shaped tail with a single spine. Adult lungworms occupy terminal bronchioles, alveolar ducts, and small pulmonary artery branches. Eggs are shed into alveoli, then hatch into first-stage larvae, ascend the airways and are swallowed and shed in the feces 5–6 weeks postinfection. Development to infective third-stage larvae occurs in intermediate hosts such as snails or slugs. Cats become infected by ingestion of the intermediate host or by ingesting paratenic hosts such as birds, rodents, amphibians, and reptiles. Third-stage larvae reach the lungs from the gastrointestinal tract *via* the circulatory system within 24 hours of ingestion.
ii. The previous history of vomiting, diarrhea, and pyrexia is suggestive of salmonellosis. *Salmonella* gastroenteritis is characterized by high fever (body temperature 40.0–41.0°C), malaise, and anorexia followed shortly by vomiting, abdominal pain, and diarrhea. Fecal shedding of *Salmonella* spp. in cats occurs for up to 6 weeks following resolution of clinical signs. Infection of the lungs most likely occurred as a result of migration of *A. abstrusus* larvae contaminated with *Salmonella* spp. during intestinal passage. Alternatively, *Salmonella* spp. bronchopneumonia may have occurred secondary to bacteremia during the acute gastroenteritis. *A. abstrusus* larvae may have liberated bacteria from walled-off granulomas during pulmonary migration.

135 A 3-year-old spayed female domestic shorthair cat was seen because of acute-onset hind-end weakness, inappetence, and lethargy of 2 days' duration (135). On physical examination, the cat was depressed and febrile (body temperature 41.5°C). It had pelvic limb ataxia, hyperesthesia over the back, renomegaly, and cloudy eyes. Blood tests showed the total protein count was 97.7 g/l, albumin was 27.7 g/l and globulins were 70 g/l, resulting in an A:G ratio of 0.39. Serum coronavirus antibody titer was 1:400. CSF was collected, and analysis revealed pleocytosis (63 leukocytes/µl) with mono-

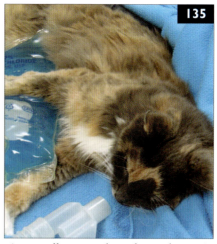

nuclear cells and neutrophils as the predominant cell type and an elevated protein concentration (1.5 g/l).

i. What are the differential diagnoses?
ii. What condition is likely to be causing the CSF findings?
iii. What therapeutic considerations should be discussed with the client?

136 A 6-month-old intact female domestic shorthair cat was presented because of coughing and tachypnea progressing over the past 24 hours. The cat lived in a colony of 15 specific pathogen-free cats. The colony was isolated from other cats, but there were other species, including pigs and dogs, in the same building. No vaccinations had been given. On physical examination, the cat had increased inspiratory effort and a crouched posture with its neck extended. There was fever (40.6°C), tachypnea (52 bpm), and decreased lung sounds over the left cranial lung field. Later in the day, six more cats were sneezing, including two with fevers and one which was coughing, but the other eight cats appeared normal. Thoracic radiographs were taken of the cat presented (136).

i. What are the differential diagnoses?
ii. What is the diagnostic plan?
iii. Are there any precautions necessary when managing this cat in the clinic?

135 i. FIP, infections with FeLV or FIV, systemic mycoses, and toxoplasmosis may present with these clinical signs, as can neurologic neoplasia, such as lymphoma. FIP meningitis and myelitis are caused by immune-complex vasculitis and a pyogranulomatous reaction.
ii. CSF findings such as these are commonly found with neurologic manifestations of FIP. Protein levels may be as high as 2 g/l, resulting in a viscous CSF.
iii. The prognosis for cats with CNS FIP is grim. Treatment protocols focus on suppression of the immune response with corticosteroids. Concurrent therapy with pentoxifylline (15 mg/kg PO q 12 h) may be considered. Its potential effects include improvement of blood flow and microcirculation, reducing neutrophil adhesion and activation, and free radical scavenging. Nutritional and fluid requirements must be addressed. This cat was euthanized as no improvement was seen with treatment, and FIP was confirmed at necropsy.

136 i. The thoracic radiographs are most consistent with bronchopneumonia. Although this unvaccinated colony is maintained in isolation, husbandry staff could bring in pathogens from outside. Since the cats are unvaccinated, they would be especially susceptible to viruses, such as FHV and FCV. However, viral infections are more likely to cause upper respiratory tract signs, although they sometimes cause pneumonia (especially in kittens), or secondary bacterial pneumonia can occur uncommonly. Another common cause of acute respiratory disease outbreaks in cats is the bacterium *Bordetella bronchiseptica*. Although the involvement of multiple cats suggests an infectious cause, certain toxic substances, particularly quaternary ammonium disinfectants, can cause similar signs.
ii. At a minimum, the diagnostic plan should include a complete blood count and thoracic radiographs. Oropharyngeal swabs should be collected for identification of FHV and FCV by PCR or viral isolation. Although the colony was previously believed to be free of retroviral infection, repeat testing for FeLV and FIV is indicated. Because this is a young, previously healthy cat with signs confined to the respiratory tract, a biochemistry panel and urinalysis may not be essential.
iii. Since this cat had not been vaccinated, it should be housed separately in the clinic, so that it neither disseminates nor acquires infectious diseases. Of the primary differential diagnoses, FCV is the most difficult to inactivate. FCV is resistant to quaternary ammonium disinfectants, but is sensitive to dilute bleach (1:32) and potassium peroxymonosulfate.

137 Case 137 is the same cat as case 136. Neutrophilia (mature neutrophils 32.8 × 10⁹/l) with a left shift (band neutrophils 2.4 × 10⁹/l) was identified on the complete blood count; FeLV and FIV tests were negative. Oropharyngeal swabs were collected for FHV and FCV isolation. Based on the clinical and radiographic findings, a BAL was performed for cytology (137) (Wrights–Giemsa stain) and culture.

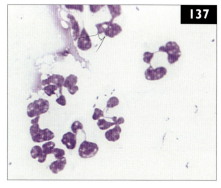

i. What is the interpretation of the BAL cytology?
ii. What is the appropriate treatment plan?
iii. How should the problem in the colony be addressed?

138 A 10-month-old intact male domestic shorthair cat was seen because of tachypnea and dyspnea, which had started suddenly 2 days previously. The cat was allowed to roam outside. Physical examination was un-remarkable apart from muffling of the heart and lung sounds on thoracic auscultation. Dorsoventral and

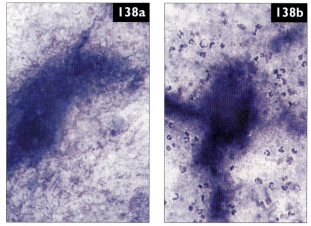

lateral radiographs were taken and showed a bilateral pleural effusion. Thoracocentesis was performed in order to remove the fluid and to make a diagnosis. A large amount of a purulent, malodorous fluid, containing small grey sulfur granules, was drained. The protein concentration in the effusion was high (57 g/l), and there was also a high leucocyte count (63 × 10⁹/l). A smear was examined cytologically at low (138a) and high magnification (138b).

i. What cell types and materials are present in the smear?
ii. What is the diagnosis?
iii. What are the recommended therapeutic procedures?

137 i. The BAL fluid is foamy and cloudy with strands of mucus. The cytospin preparation shows predominantly degenerate neutrophils, many with intracyto-plasmic bacterial rods. The tentative diagnosis is bronchopneumonia caused by the Gram-negative rod *Bordetella bronchiseptica*. BAL fluid should also be submitted for aerobic, anaerobic, and selective medium cultures for *Bordetella* spp. and *Mycoplasma* spp.

ii. In this case, treatment was initiated with enrofloxacin, intravenous fluids, and oxygen therapy. Within 36 hours, the cat was eupneic and eating well. Micro-biological evaluations revealed heavy growth of a pure culture of *B. bronchiseptica*, resistant to penicillins and cephalosporins and susceptible to fluoroquinolones. The cat was returned to the colony that day. Enrofloxacin was continued PO for a total of 3 weeks. FHV and FCV isolation were negative.

iii. By the week following the index case, 12 more cats had developed various clinical signs of fever, sneezing, nasal discharge, or coughing. Oropharyngeal swabs were collected from the entire colony, and all were positive for *B. bronchiseptica*. All cats were treated with enrofloxacin for 3 weeks. Enrofloxacin was selected for many reasons, including its long dosing interval that allowed handling of the cats only once daily, thereby reducing the risk of transmission. Other animals in the building, including dogs, pigs, and cats tested negative for *B. bronchiseptica*, and the source of the outbreak was never determined.

138 i. Cytologic examination reveals degenerating neutrophils, lymphocytes, macrophages, and some eosinophils. A population of extracellular bacteria is also seen. Moreover, the examination reveals the presence of branching, filamentous rods with beaded appearance that at high magnification appear in dense aggregates. The organisms are positive on Gram stain.

ii. The cytologic findings, in association with sulfur granules, suggest pyothorax caused by *Actinomyces* spp. or *Nocardia* spp. In doubtful cases when anaerobic and aerobic cultures are negative, acid-fast stains may help to differentiate *Nocardia* spp. (acid-fast) from *Actinomyces* spp. (not acid-fast). In this case, *Actinomyces* spp. was identified by culture.

iii. Chest drains should be placed bilaterally under general anesthesia. The tubes are sutured to the skin with nonabsorbable suture, and the pleural effusion removed by continuous or intermittent suction. Lavage of the pleural space may be performed (40 ml warmed saline q 12–24 h). Antibiotic therapy should be started pending results of microbial culture and sensitivity. This cat received chest tubes, and lavage was performed every 12 h. After 1 week, the treatment was halted because the owners decided to go no further and to euthanize the cat.

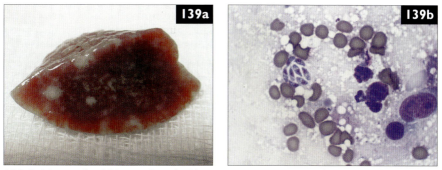

139 A 14-month-old intact female Abyssinian cat was seen after it gave birth to six healthy kittens. All kittens had been suckling shortly after birth and were observed to be healthy by the owner. However, the kittens stopped suckling and became dehydrated, icteric, and dyspneic. Three kittens died between 5 and 8 days after birth and were submitted for necropsy. Predominant changes were found in the liver (139a), and a cytologic squash was prepared from liver tissue (139b) (modified Wrights–Giemsa). Nine days after birth, the three remaining kittens were examined, and showed similar clinical signs.
i. What are the differential diagnoses for fading kitten syndrome in this litter of kittens?
ii. What diagnostic tests should be performed on the surviving kittens?
iii. What are the findings in the liver section and in the cytologic preparation?

140 A 4-year-old castrated male domestic shorthair cat was seen because of anorexia progressing over a 3-week period (140). The cat lived exclusively indoors with two other cats that appeared healthy. On physical examination the cat had an unkempt haircoat, was slightly underweight (BCS 4/9), and had mildly increased body temperature (39.3°C). Abdominal palpation revealed slightly enlarged kidneys. Complete

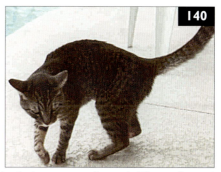

blood count, biochemistry panel, and urinalysis were performed. These showed pancytopenia, azotemia, hyperglobulinemia, mildly increased ALT activity, and inflammatory urine sediment.
i. What do the laboratory results suggest?
ii. What additional diagnostic steps are indicated?

139 i. Fading kitten syndrome has both noninfectious and infectious causes. Noninfectious causes include low birth weight, prematurity, congenital disorders, malnutrition, hypoxia/anoxia during parturition, hypothermia, maternal neglect, and neonatal isoerythrolysis (type B queen, type A sire). Infectious causes include FeLV infection, FPV infection, FIP, ascending umbilical bacterial infections (omphalophlebitis), sepsis, and neonatal toxoplasmosis. In these kittens, the most likely diagnoses are neonatal isoerythrolysis, neonatal toxoplasmosis, bacterial infection, or FIP since all may cause icterus.

ii. The queen and kittens should be blood-typed immediately and be tested for FeLV. The kittens' hematocrits should be determined to distinguish prehepatic from hepatic or posthepatic icterus. Kittens with neonatal isoerythrolysis characteristically have dark red-brown urine. Tail tip necrosis from cold-reacting IgM antibodies or thrombosis may be present. Thoracic radiographs are warranted to investigate further the kittens' dyspnea. Antibody tests for *Toxoplasma gondii* should be performed. Liver enzyme activities (e.g. ALT, ALP) are usually elevated in neonatal toxoplasmosis. However, ALP elevations in kittens are nonspecific because cats possess a bone isoenzyme of ALP. Fine-needle aspiration cytology of the liver may be useful in detecting bacterial or protozoal hepatitis.

iii. The appearance of the liver is typical of kittens infected transplacentally with *T. gondii*. There are numerous foci of white discoloration due to necrosis produced by tachyzoites. In the cytologic preparation, there is a clump of eight extracellular, banana-shaped tachyzoites amongst scattered erythrocytes. The kittens had neonatal toxoplasmosis.

140 i. These indicate that multiple organs are involved in the disease process. Together with the fever, they suggest an inflammatory (infectious or noninfectious) or neoplastic (e.g. lymphoma) condition.

ii. Thoracic and abdominal radiographs, abdominal ultrasonography, including ultrasound-guided fine-needle aspirates of the liver, kidney, and any lesions, and a bone marrow aspirate are indicated. Tests for FeLV and FIV infection should be performed.

141 Case **141** is the same cat as case **140**. Imaging revealed a mild diffuse pulmonary interstitial pattern and mild enlargement of the kidneys, liver, spleen, and mesenteric lymph nodes. Ultrasound-guided fine-needle aspirates were collected from the abnormal organs. Bone marrow was also collected for cytologic evaluation. A cytology of the kidney (**141**) (Wrights–Giemsa stain) revealed

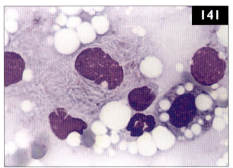

similar findings to the cytologic preparations of other organs.
i. What is the interpretation of the kidney cytology?
ii. What additional diagnostic steps are indicated?
iii. What treatment should be initiated?
iv. Are there any public health concerns?

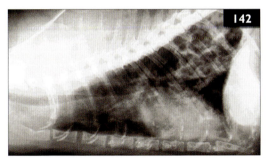

142 A 7-year-old castrated male Siamese cat was seen because of an intermittent soft cough noted for the past 6 months. The client said that the cat appeared otherwise in good health and that it was behaving normally at home. The cat was allowed outside, and had traveled extensively with its owners, including in South America. On physical examination, the respiratory rate was 48 bpm and expiratory wheezes were heard when the cat was distressed. Thoracic radiographs were taken (**142**).
i. How should the radiographic findings be described?
ii. What are the differential diagnoses suggested by these changes?
iii. What other diagnostic tests should be performed in order to achieve a definitive diagnosis?

141 i. The kidney aspirate shows macrophages containing numerous nonstaining filamentous bacteria. Similar findings were present in the liver, spleen, lymph nodes, and bone marrow. This is most consistent with disseminated mycobacteriosis.
ii. An acid-fast stain should be applied to confirm the diagnosis of mycobacteriosis. Also, a sample should be submitted for culture and sensitivity. Disseminated mycobacteriosis is usually diagnosed where there is decreased immune function. Further tests could include tests to confirm the FeLV- and FIV-free status of the cat, lymphocyte subset analysis, serum immunoglobulin concentrations, and phagocyte function tests. In this case, flow cytometric analysis showed a severe decrease in CD4+ lymphocytes, implying there was a significant decrease in cell-mediated immunity. *Mycobacterium xenopi* was diagnosed by culture of the bone marrow; this is a saprophytic opportunistic organism infrequently associated with disseminated mycobacteriosis.
iii. Initial therapy should include IV fluid therapy for diuresis and nutritional support. Treatment of disseminated mycobacteriosis in immunodeficient patients requires the long-term (possibly life-long) administration of multiple antibiotics. In this case, pending culture results, treatment was initiated with clarithromycin, enrofloxacin, and clofazamine. Sensitivity testing confirmed these were appropriate selections. The cat was still alive 4 years after the original diagnosis.
iv. Because saprophytic opportunistic mycobacterial organisms are widely distributed in soil and water and are not readily transmitted among individuals, infected patients are not considered to pose a zoonotic threat.

142 i. The most prominent changes on the radiographs are the patchy interstitial infiltrates.
ii. These nonspecific changes suggest inflammation caused by immune reaction (e.g. hypersensitivity, asthma). When nodules or a regional difference in density is seen, chronic lungworm or fluke infection, fungal granulomas, or neoplasia may be added as considerations. Heart failure leading to pulmonary edema is considered less likely, as cardiac silhouette and vessel size are normal.
iii. Fecal examination should be performed in an attempt to detect lungworm ova or larvae or fluke ova. If negative, then tracheal wash or bronchoalveolar lavage fluid should be collected for fluid cytology evaluation in the absence of cardiac disease. In this case, a mixture of inflammatory cells (neutrophils and eosinophils predominating) on cytologic assessment suggested allergic or parasitic small airway disease. Less commonly, neoplastic and fungal conditions are associated with increased numbers of eosinophils. Eggs or larvae may be seen on cytology.

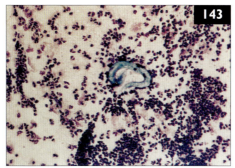

143 Case **143** is the same cat as case **142**. A parasite was recovered on tracheal washing (**143**).
i. What is this organism?
ii. How do cats become infected with these parasites?
iii. What is the recommended treatment?

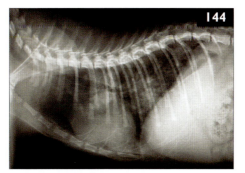

144 A young adult intact male stray domestic shorthair cat recently adopted by a new owner was seen because of cough and dyspnea. Since it was found 3 weeks earlier, it had had a reduced appetite and had not gained weight. On physical examination, the body temperature was normal. The cat was slightly dyspneic with inspiratory and expiratory crackles over all of the lung fields on auscultation. No nasal discharge or sneezing was observed. A complete blood count was performed and showed moderate eosinophilia. Thoracic radiographs were taken (**144**).
i. What is the most likely explanation for the clinical, hematologic, and radiographic changes in this cat?
ii. What further diagnostic tests should be recommended?
iii. How should the cat be treated?
iv. If there are other animals in the household, how high is the potential risk for transmission of the disease?

143 i. This organism is the lungworm *Aelurostrongylus abstrusus*.
ii. Cats are the terminal host for three different types of lung parasite: (1) *A. abstrusus* infections are often subclinical and self-limiting. The intermediate host is a terrestrial snail or slug. Eggs are deposited in alveoli where they hatch and release larvae, which are swallowed and shed in feces. These larvae may best be demonstrated using Baermann fecal filtration. Because eggs are shed intermittently, multiple fecal samples may need to be examined. (2) *Paragonimus kellicotti* is a lung fluke with two sequential intermediary hosts: an amphibious snail and a crayfish. Immature flukes form cystic cavities within the lungs. Thus, cats with *P. kellicotti* may have severe dyspnea or, more commonly, chronic cough. Sedimentation techniques are the best way to demonstrate fluke ova in feces. (3) *Eucoleus aerophila* (previously *Capillaria aerophila*) has a direct life cycle; however, earthworms and rodents may be a source of infective ova for cats. The white, thread-like adult worms live in the trachea and bronchi. Although most cases are asymptomatic, a persistent dry cough may occur and may be elicited by tracheal palpation. Radiographic signs are less likely than with the other two parasites because of the agent's localization.
iii. The most commonly recommended treatment for lungworm infection is fenbendazole (50 mg/kg PO q 24 h for 12–20 days).

144 i. This cat may have a lungworm infestation. The commonest lungworm in cats is *Aelurostrongylus abstrusus*, which can be detected in up to 39% of stray cats. The adult nematode lives in alveoli and terminal bronchioles, causing bronchopneumonia. Clinical signs develop if the worm burden is high; many cats with mild infection do not show them. Thoracic radiographs typically demonstrate bronchointerstitial and patchy alveolar infiltrates, as in this case. Many cats have peripheral eosinophilia.
   Other differential diagnoses are bronchial asthma and dirofilariasis.
ii. Fecal testing should be performed, using either Baermann fecal examination or zinc sulfate flotation, to look for *A. abstrusus* eggs. Another option is to demonstrate the larvae in a BAL sample. This is especially helpful if a Baermann filtration is negative in a cat with suspected infestation, since larvae are shed only intermittently.
   The patient should also be tested for FeLV and FIV.
iii. In cats with mild infection, the disease is usually self-limiting. If clinical signs are present, as in this case, cats should be treated once the diagnosis has been established. One treatment option with few side-effects is fenbendazole.
iv. Cats can become infested if they ingest the intermediate host directly (snails and slugs), or if they eat animals that have been feeding on them. Thus, direct transmission of the disease to other pets is impossible.

145 A 7-year-old castrated male domestic shorthair cat was seen because of a gradually developing stiffness in the left front limb. The cat was an indoor/outdoor cat. It was otherwise healthy. No pain was apparent, and the cat did not withdraw the limb in response to pinch. Radiographs of the limb were normal. The initial recommendation was to observe the cat at home. However, on physical examination 1 week later, the contralateral limb was affected, and the facial expression was abnormal. The ears were erect, the lips were drawn back, the forehead was creased, jaw tone was increased, and there was ptylism.
i. What infectious agent is suggested by these findings?
ii. How is the diagnosis made?
iii. What treatment is recommended, and what prognosis should be given?

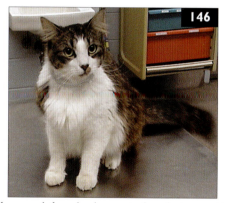

146 A 9-month-old spayed female domestic longhair cat (**146**) was seen for a consultation. The cat lived in a single-cat household in a rural area and was allowed to go outside. It was healthy and had received its primary vaccination series (FPV, FHV, FCV, FeLV, rabies). The owner had had a kidney transplant 2 weeks earlier and was now on high-dose immunosuppressive therapy. She had brought her cat so that it could be checked for any potential zoonotic infections (e.g. toxoplasmosis) it was carrying that might pose a threat to her. Physical examination was unremarkable; however, some flea feces were found on the hair coat. The cat had a *Toxoplasma gondii* IgG antibody titer of 1:1024 (high titer) and an IgM antibody titer of 1:512 (moderate titer).
i. How should the *T. gondii* antibody titer be interpreted?
ii. Is the cat a risk for the immunosuppressed owner?
iii. For which other infection should tests be performed?

145 i. The clinical signs are consistent with tetanus, caused by the Gram-positive anerobic bacterium *Clostridium tetani*. Rabies is also a consideration, but the week-long slowly progressive and localized course makes rabies less likely.

ii. Cats with tetanus may or may not have a history of a noticeable wound in the area of the original clinical signs. Clinical signs of increased muscle tone and altered facial expression are characteristic of tetanus. Other than muscle spasm-induced elevations in the muscle enzymes, e.g. creatine kinase (CK), aspartate transaminase (AST) and wound-related leukocytosis, there are no abnormalities in the complete blood count, biochemistry profile, and urinalysis. The presence of antibodies to tetanus toxin in the blood, when compared to a control animal, substantiates the diagnosis. Muscle biopsy results are generally unremarkable other than showing evidence of muscle trauma. Isolation of the organism is difficult.

iii. Because cats are relatively resistant to *C. tetani*, they usually only develop localized tetanus. Thus, treatment with antitoxin may not be used. Besides the use of antibiotics (e.g. penicillin G), given both IV and IM close to the wound site, sedatives may be helpful in reducing spasms. Combinations of chlorpromazine and phenobarbital have been used; alternatively, diazepam or midazolam may control spasms and excitability. Most cats have reversible disease. Cats with localized tetanus have a more favorable prognosis than those with rapidly progressive generalized disease.

146 i. As demonstrated by the high IgG titer, the cat had been infected with *Toxoplasma gondii* at least 3 weeks previously (as IgG antibodies take at least 3 weeks to rise), but probably much longer ago. This has resulted in a latent infestation that may be reactivated later in life, usually after immunosuppression. Only newly-infested cats shed *T. gondii* in their feces for about 10 days. Thus, a healthy cat that has *T. gondii* IgG antibodies is not a risk for the owner and will never be a risk.

ii. Given the statements above, it is clear that this cat is not a risk for its immunosuppressed owner. Epidemiologic tests suggest that eating undercooked or raw meat (in which *T. gondii* cysts may persist) plays a greater role in the risk of human infection than contact with cats.

iii. As the cat has fleas, tests for *Bartonella* spp. infection should be performed. It is prudent to discuss the advantages and disadvantages of *Bartonella* spp. testing with each individual cat owner and document the outcome of the discussion in the medical record.

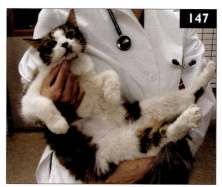

147 Case 147 is the same cat as case 146 (147). Antibody tests for *Bartonella henselae* and *B. clarridgeiae* were performed and the cat had a *B. henselae* titer of 1:1024 (high titer).
i. How should the positive *B. henselae* test be interpreted?
ii. What diseases can be caused by *B. henselae* and *B. clarridgeiae* in people and in cats?
iii. How are *Bartonella* spp. transmitted?
iv. Should the cat's infection be treated?

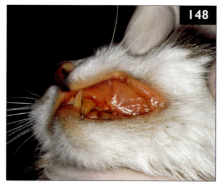

148 A 5-month-old neutered male domestic shorthair cat was seen because of ascites, icterus (148), and fever. The cat came from a shelter that housed 127 cats at that time. Cats were kept in groups of 10–20. The cat was in very poor condition and was euthanized. Necropsy examination confirmed the diagnosis of FIP.
i. If FIP is a problem in a shelter, what should be recommended?
ii. Is FIP vaccination useful in this situation?
iii. Under what other circumstances should vaccination be recommended?

147 i. The cat has antibodies against *B. henselae*; this is consistent with *B. henselae* infection. As the cat is infected, there is a zoonotic concern for an immuno-suppressed owner.

ii. Both *B. henselae* and *B. clarridgeiae* can cause cat-scratch disease (CSD) in people, a relatively harmless disease. However, immunosuppressed people may develop more serious diseases when infected, including parenchymal peliosis, bacillary angiomatosis, endocarditis, neuroretinitis, and oculoglandular syndrome. Most cats infected naturally with *Bartonella* spp. have no clinical signs.

iii. Transmission from cat to cat usually occurs *via* fleas. *Bartonella* spp. live inside red blood cells (without causing anemia). Fleas ingest these while sucking blood, and transmit the infection to another cat in the same way. Fleas digest the the blood containing the *Bartonella* spp. and the living bacteria will be present in flea feces. The cat will get the flea feces under its claws while scratching itself. If they scratch someone and the claws penetrate the skin, *Bartonella* spp. may be transmitted. It has been shown that bacteremia is much more likely in cats <1 year old than in older ones thus, young cats are more likely to transmit the infection.

iv. As the cat is young and has fleas, and the owner is severely immunosuppressed, the cat should be treated with doxycycline for 3 weeks. Doxycycline will not eliminate infection, but it will significantly reduce the bacterial load. In addition, good flea control and keeping the cat indoors are essential. Declawing has not been shown to prevent transmission and is not recommended.

148 i. Prevention of FIP in a shelter situation is virtually impossible unless cats are strictly kept in separate cages and handled only with barrier precautions (comparable to isolation units). Isolation is often not effective because of the ease with which FCoV is transported on clothes, shoes, dust, and cats. Adopters should understand that FCoV is unavoidable in multiple-cat environments, and that FIP is an unavoidable consequence of endemic FCoV. Shelters should ensure facilities can be cleaned easily to minimize virus spread.

ii. A MLV intranasal FIP vaccine is available in many countries. However, the true efficacy of this vaccine is controversial; vaccination in an FCoV-endemic environ-ment or in households with known cases of FIP is not expected to be effective.

iii. Vaccination might be of some benefit in cats that live in households with a small number of cats without previous FCoV exposure. As the vaccine is ineffective when cats have already been exposed to FCoV, antibody testing may be beneficial before vaccination. The vaccine is at least safe and does not induce antibody-dependent enhancement of FIP but its efficacy is debated.

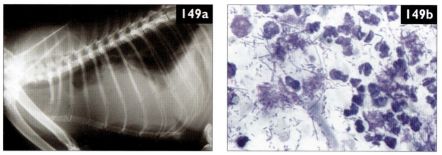

149 A 5-year-old castrated male domestic shorthair cat was seen because of a 7-day history of anorexia, dyspnea, and lethargy. On physical examination, the cat had marked inspiratory dyspnea, an increased respiratory rate (50 bpm), and a high body temperature (39.7°C). The heart sounds were muffled. Thoracic radiographs were taken (149a). A sample of pleural fluid was aspirated (149b) (modified Wrights–Giemsa).
i. What are the three most likely diagnoses based on the radiograph?
ii. What does the cytology of the pleural fluid show, and is it typical for this disease?
iii. By what mechanisms can this disease occur in cats?

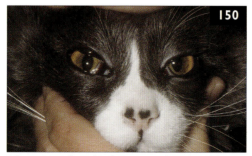

150 A five-year-old castrated male domestic shorthair cat was seen because of lethargy of 2 days' duration. The cat was kept both indoors and outdoors and was current on vaccinations. On physical examination, the cat had pale mucous membranes, tachycardia (220 bpm), and bilateral scleral hemorrhages (150).
i. What are the differential diagnoses?
ii. What is the diagnostic plan?

149 i. There is a large volume of pleural fluid within the thorax, elevating the trachea dorsally and displacing the carina caudally. It is not possible to rule out the presence of a cranial mediastinal mass on the lateral view. Pyothorax, FIP, or cranial mediastinal lymphoma is the most likely cause in this cat.

ii. The pleural fluid shows many degenerate neutrophils and masses of pleomorphic bacteria, including long filamentous bacteria and bacilli. Therefore, the cat had pyothorax. Most cases of feline pyothorax are polymicrobial infections of obligate anaerobic and facultative bacteria, similar in composition to the bacterial flora of the healthy feline oropharynx. These bacteria include *Bacteroides* spp., *Fusobacterium* spp., *Peptostreptococcus* spp., *Clostridium* spp., *Actinomyces* spp., *Eubacterium* spp., *Propionibacterium* spp., *Pasteurella multocida*, *Prevotella* spp., *Porphyromonas* spp., *Escherichia coli*, *Staphylococcus* spp., *Streptococcus* spp., and *Mycoplasma* spp. Occasionally, fungi may cause pyothorax (e.g. *Candida* spp., *Cryptococcus* spp., *Blastomyces* spp.).

iii. Infection of the pleural space may occur *via* hematogenous (e.g. systemic sepsis) or lymphatic spread, extension from an adjacent structure (e.g. bronchopneumonia, parapneumonic spread, esophageal rupture, mediastinitis, subphrenic infection), or by direct inoculation (e.g. penetrating trauma, foreign body, thoracocentesis, thoracic surgery). However, the mechanism of pleural space infection is often not identified.

150 i. Scleral hemorrhage is the most significant finding. The most likely causes are head trauma or a clotting disorder.

ii. The initial evaluation should include a complete blood count, biochemical panel, urinalysis, platelet count, prothrombin time (PT), partial thromboplastin time (PTT), fibrin degradation products (FDPs), and tests for FeLV and FIV. A cystocentesis or other invasive procedures should not be performed until the clotting parameters have been assessed.

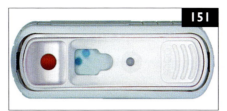

151 Case 151 is the same cat as case 150. The cat was positive for FeLV antigen and negative for FIV antibodies (151). The PT (7 sec), PTT (13 sec), and FDPs (20 µg/ml) were within the reference interval.

Blood profile/biochemistry panel	Results
Hematocrit	0.21 l/l
RBC	4.0×10^{12}/l
Platelets	18×10^{9}/l
Hemoglobin	4.2 mmol/l
Total protein	45 g/l
Albumin	21 g/l
Globulins	24 g/l
Urinalysis (voided sample)	
Protein	+

i. What is the interpretation of the laboratory values?
ii. Are any other diagnostic procedures indicated?

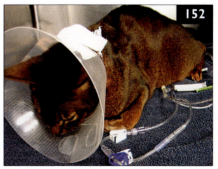

152 A 2-year-old spayed female Abyssinian cat from Vancouver, Canada, was seen because of concern over a 3-day history of cough, progressive lethargy, and inappetence (152). On physical examination, weight loss was evident. The cat was tachypneic (respiratory rate 56 bpm), had diffuse harsh bronchovesicular sounds on thoracic auscultation, and had a moist cough during examination. Body temperature was elevated at 40.3°C. Blood pressure was 150 mmHg systolic.
i. What diagnostic tests are appropriate?
ii. Is there a zoonotic risk?

151 i. There is anemia and panhypoproteinemia, which are suggestive of blood loss. Severe thrombocytopenia with normal coagulation parameters suggests a clotting disorder due to platelet deficiency. The cat is positive for FeLV antigen. FeLV infection is the most common cause of thrombocytopenia in cats.

ii. A thorough evaluation with imaging and bone marrow cytology should be performed to rule out any complicating conditions such as lymphoma or bone marrow failure. In this case, bone marrow evaluation revealed a hypercellular marrow with increased megakaryocytes suggestive of abnormal thrombopoiesis or immune destruction of platelets. Melena was observed the following day, suggesting that a major site of blood loss was the gastrointestinal tract. Some cats with FeLV-associated thrombocytopenia respond to immunosuppressive dosages of prednisolone. The cat was discharged with prednisolone (2 mg/kg PO q 24 h). At re-evaluation 2 weeks later, the platelets had increased to 78,000/µl and the hematocrit had increased to 0.27 l/l.

152 i. The following tests should be performed: (1) radiographs, (2) a complete blood count, biochemical panel, and urinalysis, (3) FeLV and FIV tests, and (4) fecal sedimentation and flotation.

These should also be considered: (1) tests for *Toxoplasma gondii*, (2) tests for heartworm infection, and (3) a bronchial wash for cytology and culture (if the cat is stable enough).

In this case, radiographs showed a diffuse interstitial to alveolar pattern and a small pleural effusion. The cat had a *T. gondii* IgM antibody titer of 1:1024 (high) and a *T. gondii* IgG antibody titer of 1:1024 (high). Both high IgM and IgG titers can be present in toxoplasma asymptomatic cats; thus, further diagnostic tests are indicated. Treatment with clindamycin or trimethoprim/sulfonamide should nevertheless be initiated. Clinical signs may worsen early in therapy, as dying organisms stimulate additional inflammation. Sometimes, treatment with anti-inflammatory doses of corticosteroids is necessary. There should be a response within a few days.

ii. Infection with *T. gondii* during pregnancy in women occurs from infection with oocysts from cats' feces, which must be in the environment for 24 hours or more before they are infective. Hence, scooping the litter box twice a day prevents the risk of oocyte infectivity. Veterinary staff who handle cats do not have a higher prevalence of serum IgG reactivity. Also, once a cat has mounted an immune response and has *T. gondii* IgG antibodies it does not shed *T. gondii* and is not a risk to people.

153 A 9-year-old neutered male domestic shorthair cat from Florida, USA, was seen because of chronic nasal congestion unresponsive to antibiotics for 6 months. On physical examination, there was inspiratory stertor and bilateral mucopurulent nasal discharge. A 3 mm hairless nodule was present on the bridge of the nose (153a), and a similar lesion was present on the right metacarpal pad. The left globe was deviated slightly laterally.

What is an appropriate diagnostic plan to address the chronic nasal discharge and the skin lesions?

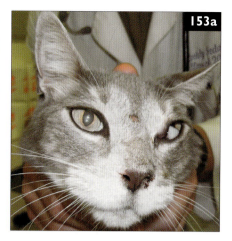

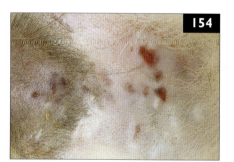

154 A 5-year-old neutered male domestic shorthair cat was seen because of chronic, nonhealing lesions on the ventral abdomen. It was allowed to roam outside. A veterinarian had performed punch biopsies in which pyogranulomatous inflammation was found. However, no microorganisms were seen. The cat had been treated with amoxicillin/clavulanate, but there had been no response. On presentation, the cat was bright, alert, and responsive. Multiple deep cutaneous and subcutaneous nonpainful nodules of variable size and ulceration were found on the ventral abdomen and inguinal area (154).

i. What are the potential reasons why the biopsy was not conclusive?
ii. What are the most likely differential diagnoses?

153 A complete blood count, biochemical panel, urinalysis, tests for FeLV and FIV, and thoracic radiography should be performed. They were all unremarkable. A CT scan showed a mass in the left nasal cavity invading the left retro-orbital space, crossing the septum to the right nasal cavity, and impinging on the cribriform plate. Fine-needle aspirates and biopsies were collected from the cutaneous lesions, the left nasal mass, and the retro-orbital mass.

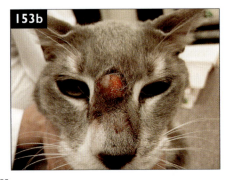

Aspirates of the cutaneous lesions suggested protothecosis, whereas aspirates from the left nasal and retro-orbital masses showed large-cell lymphoma. Biopsies confirmed the cytologic findings, and culture of tissues from the cutaneous lesions produced a pure culture of *Prototheca wickerhammii* sensitive to itraconazole and clotrimazole. Imaging of the abdomen is indicated to evaluate for systemic involvement of either disease.

Feline protothecosis is limited to cutaneous forms. In this cat, treatment was initiated with oral itraconazole and topical clotrimazole. Nasal lymphosarcoma is highly responsive to radiotherapy, which was recommended to avoid immunosuppression from chemotherapy. The owner elected chemotherapy, however, and the cat was treated with prednisolone, vincristine, and cyclophosphamide. Clinical remission was complete, with restoration of normal facial structure, within 7 days. The protothecosis lesions, however, did not respond to treatment and gradually enlarged (153b), but did not bother the cat. It was euthanized 8 months later, however, when the lymphoma came out of remission.

154 i. The main lesion is located in the subcutaneous fat tissue within granulation tissue. This is usually too deep for sampling specimens through punch biopsies. An excisional or, at least, deep wedge biopsy of such lesions is strongly recommended. Special stains such as Giemsa, PAS, GMS, and acid-fast stains are always indicated in pyogranulomatous lesions because the microorganisms can be easily overlooked with a routine H&E stain.
ii. The major differential diagnoses are: (1) Deep bacterial infections, including opportunistic mycobacteriosis, nocardiosis, actinomycosis, and bacterial pseudomycetoma. (2) Deep fungal infections, including phaeohyphomycosis, cryptococcosis, histoplasmosis, and blastomycosis. (3) Algae, including pythiosis. (4) Noninfectious diseases, including idiopathic panniculitis or foreign-body reaction.

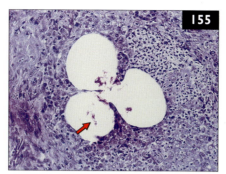

155 Case 155 is the same cat as case 154. It was decided to repeat taking skin biopsies and to request an acid-fast stain. Histopathology showed a pyogranulomatous dermatitis and panniculitis with central clear zones containing acid-fast positive filamentous organisms (155, arrow) (acid-fast stain).
i. What is the tentative diagnosis?
ii. Which additional tests could be performed to identity the organisms?
iii. What are the treatment recommendations and the prognosis for this disease?

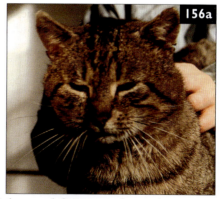

156 A 4-year-old castrated male domestic shorthair cat (156a) was seen after being in a fight and developing a small draining abscess on the dorsum of its head. The cat became lethargic and obtunded 5 days later and was observed to be head pressing. The cat lived mainly outdoors in Sydney, Australia. On physical examination, the cat had a high body temperature (39.8°C). The menace response was absent in the right eye and postural reactions were diminished in the right forelimb and right hind limb. Spinal reflexes were normal, and no cranial nerve deficits were detected.
i. What is the neuroanatomical localization of the lesion?
ii. What are the differential diagnoses?
iii. How should this case be further investigated?

155 i. The diagnosis is mycobacteriosis. *Nocardia* spp. stain partially with acid-fast stain as well, and can sometimes be difficult to differentiate from *Mycobacteria* spp.
ii. Mycobacterial culture and sensitivity and PCR assay are the most effective tests for the identification of the organism. However, culture and sensitivity testing is essential for determining appropriate antimicrobial treatment.
iii. Treatment is often complicated by chronicity, variable severity, poor response to therapy, and lack of early diagnosis. If cultures are still pending, treatment should be started with one or, preferably, two to three different oral antibiotics. Currently, clarithromycin is the antibiotic of choice. Once the susceptibility test results are available, an alternative may be needed. Other antibiotics that are effective are doxycycline, enrofloxacin, ciprofloxacin, and clofazimine. It is recommended to use high doses of these for 3–12 months, and antibiotics should be given for 1–2 months after complete clinical cure. Wide surgical excision, in conjunction with systemic antimicrobial therapy, is often necessary. It is recommended, however, to start systemic antibiotic therapy at least 1 month before surgery, thereby enabling the lesion to regress first. The prognosis is good if the cat is managed properly. Side-effects of long-term therapy may occur and are specific to the drugs selected.

156 i. The cat has a left forebrain lesion as indicated by contralateral postural re-action and menace deficits, decreased mentation, and head pressing.
ii. An epidural, subdural, or subarachnoid abscess causing pressure on cerebral parenchyma or an abscess of the cerebrum itself secondary to a penetrating cat-bite wound is the most likely diagnosis. Differential diagnoses include neoplasia (e.g. lymphoma), hemorrhage secondary to trauma or generalized clotting disorder, FIP, mycotic granuloma, toxoplasmosis, or aberrant parasitic migration.
iii. The cat should be tested for FeLV and FIV since both viruses are associated with lymphomagenesis. A complete blood count should be performed to evaluate for cytopenias suggestive of FeLV or FIV infection or an inflammatory leukogram supporting a cat-bite abscess. Radiographs may localize a deficit in the skull where penetrating trauma from a cat bite occurred. Ideally, advanced imaging (MRI) should be performed to delineate the area of the abscess. If this is not available immediately, the area of the penetrating cat bite should be surgically explored to establish drainage of the abscess. Unfortunately, the owner elected euthanasia in this case. The abscess was subdural (**156b**, arrow).

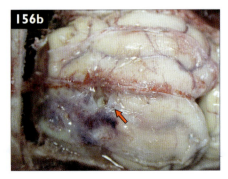

156b

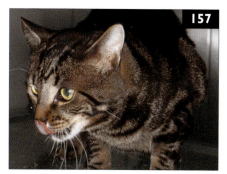

157 A 10-year-old spayed female domestic shorthair cat (157) was seen for its annual wellness visit. The cat had tested FIV-positive at 5 years of age when it was seen because of a bite wound. Since that time, the cat had been kept indoors only. The annual wellness visit included a complete blood count, biochemistry panel (both unremarkable), and urinalysis.

Urinalysis (cystocentesis)	Results
Color/appearance	yellow, clear
Specific gravity	1.035
pH	6.0
Protein	++++
Glucose	–
Ketone	–
Bilirubin	–
Blood	+
RBC	5–10 cells/hpf
WBC	<3 cells/hpf
Casts	0 cells/hpf

i. What is the interpretation of the urinalysis?
ii. What are the rule-outs for this problem and the underlying pathophysiologic mechanisms?

158 Case 158 is the same cat as case 157. The cat had glomerulonephritis secondary to FIV infection. A repeat FIV test confirmed the infection (158).

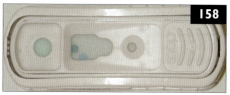

i. What is the next diagnostic step?
ii. What are the major consequences of this problem?
iii. How should the cat be treated?

157 i. The cat has proteinuria.

ii. The differentials for proteinuria are preglomerular, glomerular, and postglomerular proteinuria. Most commonly, the urine is contaminated with protein 'after' the glomerulus (postglomerular). *Preglomerular proteinuria* is rare and is caused by excessive production of small molecular weight proteins (e.g. Bence Jones proteins), by neoplastic plasma cells (e.g. multiple myeloma, plasmocytoma) or, rarely, excessive release of hemoglobin and myoglobin from damaged red blood cells and muscle tissue. *Glomerular proteinuria* can be either transient ('physiologic proteinuria'), without primary changes in the kidneys or persistent ('pathologic proteinuria'), with detectable morphologic changes. 'Physiologic proteinuria', also called 'pseudo-proteinuria', 'benign proteinuria', 'reversible proteinuria', or 'proteinuria without morphologic changes', is transient, and abates when the underlying cause is corrected. Strenuous exercise, seizures, pyrexia, exposure to extreme heat or cold, and stress are examples of conditions that may cause physiologic proteinuria. In cats, the most common reasons for transient proteinuria are stress and pyrexia. *Pathologic glomerular proteinuria* is nonreversible and is associated with morphologic changes in the kidneys. It is caused by glomerulonephritis or, rarely, amyloidosis. In this cat, the sediment was free of inflammation. There was a small amount of blood, but not enough to explain the 4+ protein. Thus, this cat has glomerular proteinuria, most likely due to glomerulonephritis as a consequence of its FIV infection.

158 i. The urine protein excretion should be quantified, to evaluate the severity of renal lesions as well as the response to treatment or the progression of disease. Today, the most commonly used method is the urine protein to creatinine ratio (UPC). This ratio negates the effects of urine concentration on the protein concentration. A UPC of <0.5 is considered normal in cats.

ii. Glomerular disease associated with protein loss has three major consequences. First, the significant loss of albumin causes a decrease in plasma oncotic pressure, leading to formation of edema and/or ascites, and muscle wasting. The second serious consquence is the loss of antithrombin III. This leads to hypercoagulability and an increased risk of thromboembolic disease. The third major consequence is the development of secondary renal tubular damage. Persistent proteinuria leads to damage of the tubular epithelium, resulting in renal failure. If one of these three consequences occurs, the prognosis becomes guarded.

iii. Symptomatic treatment should be instituted. An ACE inhibitor (e.g. benazepril) should be given to reduce the amount of protein in the urine, thus reducing the severity of the tubular damage. Also, ω3-fatty acids may be beneficial in preventing further glomerular damage. In addition, the cat should be started on a slightly protein-reduced diet to slow the progression of renal disease.

159 A 10-year-old spayed female domestic shorthair cat was seen because of renomegaly that had been diagnosed by a referring veterinarian. Both kidneys were extremely enlarged; this could be seen on physical examination (159a) as well as on the radiographs (159b). Values of complete blood count, biochemistry panel, and urinalysis were all within the reference intervals. Cytology of the kidneys was diagnostic of lymphoma, and the cat was positive in a FeLV antigen test. The owner did not want to use antitumor chemotherapy; she only wanted to try alternative treatment or immunomodulatory drugs against the FeLV infection.

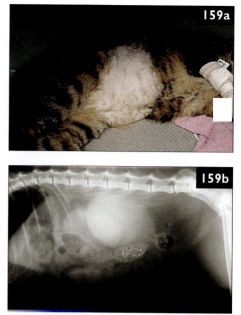

i. How do immunomodulatory drugs work?

ii. Do they have any effect in FeLV-infected cats?

160 A 4-year-old intact male domestic longhair cat was seen with a 4-week history of lethargy, anorexia, generalized seizures, hindleg weakness, and circular raised lesions on the face and back. The cat lived indoors/outdoors in a rural area. It had been vaccinated

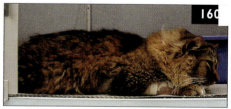

against FPV, FHV, FCV, FeLV, and rabies, and was negative for FIV and FeLV. Recent testing showed mild hyperglycemia, hypercalcemia, and urinary leukocytosis. On presentation, it was lethargic and recumbent (160). Red, firm skin nodules were noted on the head and flank. There was generalized lymph node enlargement. Neurologic examination showed a stuporous cat with nonambulatory upper motor neuron tetraparesis and normal to hyperactive spinal reflexes. Postural reactions were decreased on the right and absent on the left side. Cranial nerve examination showed absent menace response of the left eye, waxing and waning constriction and dilation of the pupils, and decreased response to sensory stimuli on the right nostril.

i. What is the neuroanatomical localization of the neurologic findings?

ii. What are the differential diagnoses?

159 i. It has been suggested that immunomodulators may benefit infected animals by restoring compromised immune function, thereby allowing them to control viral burden and recover. Most of the reports are difficult to interpret due to lack of placebo control groups, small numbers of cats used, and additional supportive treatments given.

ii. Controlled studies including large numbers of naturally FeLV-infected cats are lacking and, if performed, they mostly failed to show a beneficial effect. Studies have been published using a number of 'immunomodulators', including 'paramunity' inducers pind-avi (*Parapoxvirus avis*) and pind-orf (*Parapoxvirus ovis*), acemannan, a carbohydrate polymer from the *aloe vera* plant, *Staphylococcus* protein A (SPA), *Propionibacterium acnes* (formerly *Corynebacterium parvum*), Bacille Calmette–Guérin (BCG), *Serratia marcescens*, levamisole, and diethylcarbamazine. Scientific data do not support the use of immunomodulatory therapy in FeLV-infected cats. This cat was treated with SPA, but had to be euthanized 4 weeks later due to progression to renal failure associated with the renal lymphoma.

160 i. Stupor can be due to metabolic, toxic, or intracranial causes. Taken together, the neurologic signs are best explained by multifocal intracranial disease (forebrain and brainstem). Seizures, decreased response to stimulation of the nostril, and decreased menace response suggest forebrain disease. Cats with forebrain disease will usually still be ambulatory. Nonambulatory upper motor neuron tetraparesis suggests brainstem or cervical spinal cord (C1–C5) disease. The pupillary abnormalities are most suggestive of retinal, optic nerve, or chiasm disease, and an ophthalmic examination should, therefore, be performed to exclude intraocular disease.

ii. Inflammatory disease is the most likely differential for progressive multifocal intracranial disease in a young adult cat. This suspicion is further supported by results of ophthalmic examination demonstrating exudative granulomatous retinitis. Hypercalcemia can be associated with granulomatous disease as well. The mild hyperglycemia in the absence of glucosuria is suggestive of a stress response. Normal body temperature and normal blood leukocytes do not exclude the possibility of meningoencephalitis. Here, a few leukocytes in the urine, skin lesions, and enlarged peripheral lymph nodes were the only extraneural signs of inflammation. Frequent causes of meningoencephalitis in the cat are FIP, non-FIP viral encephalitis, toxoplasmosis, bacterial encephalitis arising from the sinuses, chronic otitis media/ interna, or bites, *Cuterebra* larva migrans, and cryptococcosis. Cryptococcosis frequently causes cutaneous nodules, nasal disease, retinitis, optic neuritis, and meningoencephalitis in the cat. Other differentials besides inflammatory disease would be hydrocephalus, metabolic, toxic, or nutritional encephalopathy (hepatic encephalopathy, thiamine deficiency, lead poisoning), and neoplasia.

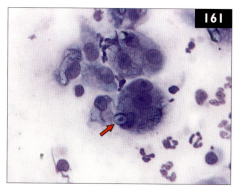

161 Case 161 is the same cat as case 160. A cytologic impression was prepared with Romanowsky stain from the red, firm skin nodules (161). These demonstrated capsulated yeasts (arrow).

The histopathologic report of the skin biopsy (from the same area) described a well-circumscribed accumulation of round thickly encapsulated yeasts forming a nodule within the dermis and extending to the subcutaneous fat. Few lymphocytes, plasma cells, and neutrophils were seen.

i. What other diagnostic procedure should be performed to identify the yeasts?
ii. What are the treatment options?

162 A 6-year-old spayed female domestic shorthair cat was seen because of anorexia, and it had a large number of small disseminated cutaneous nodules and an ulcerated swelling on the left forelimb (162). There were also two conjunctival lesions in the left eye. The cat lived mainly outdoors in Turin, Italy. On physical examination, the cat had a high body temperature (40.5°C), and was depressed. The ocular examination revealed bilateral chorioretinitis.

i. What are the differential diagnoses for this cat's problems?
ii. How should the diagnosis be confirmed?

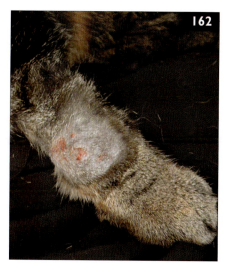

161 i. The yeast-like organisms seen were suggestive of cryptococcosis. Cryptococcosis may be confirmed with cryptococcal antigen testing by latex agglutination, which is highly sensitive and specific and can be performed with serum and CSF. The cryptococcal latex antigen titer in this case was 1:65536 (extremely high). If CSF analysis is considered as a means of diagnosing cryptococcal meningoencephalitis, precautions should be taken to avoid inadvertent brain herniation and respiratory arrest due to raised intracranial pressure. Intubation, hyperventilation and pretreatment with mannitol are recommended, and only a minimal amount of CSF should be removed. Most cats with cryptococcosis have detectable antigen in serum and, thus, CSF puncture can usually be avoided.

ii. Treatment options include fluconazole, itraconazole, ketoconazole, and amphotericin B. Fluconazole and itraconazole are the most widely-used treatments for cryptococcosis in cats due to their lower cost, ease of application, and fewer side-effects like anorexia, vomiting, and hepatic disease. For CNS infections, fluconazole may be the drug of choice because of its better penetration into the CNS. Amphotericin B requires frequent hospital visits because it must be given parenterally and can be nephrotoxic. Antifungal treatment should be continued for at least 1–2 months after clinical resolution.

162 i. The problems are fever, disseminated cutaneous nodules, nodular conjunctival lesions, bilateral chorioretinitis, and forelimb swelling. The differential diagnoses include various systemic, mainly infectious diseases based on the region where the cat lives. This is particularly true for fungal diseases or atypical infections (e.g. leishmaniasis, babesiosis). Common causes of feline chorioretinitis include FeLV infection, FIV infection, FIP, *Toxoplasma gondii* infection, and fungal infections (e.g. *Cryptococcus* spp., *Histoplasma capsulatum*). Recently, FHV infection and *Bartonella* spp. infection have also been implicated as possible causes of posterior uveitis. The skin lesions could be associated with feline leishmaniasis, fungal infection, atypical mycobacteriosis, algal infection, and neoplasia (e.g. lymphoma).

ii. A complete blood count, biochemical profile, urinalysis, and FeLV and FIV tests are indicated, as are radiographs of the thorax and affected forelimb and fine-needle aspirates of cutaneous and forelimb lesions. Bilateral chorioretinitis suggests fungal diseases, FIP, or toxoplasmosis. Analysis of aqueous humor may be helpful in achieving a diagnosis.

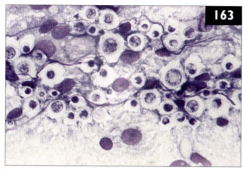

163 Case 163 is the same cat as case 162. Radiographs of the left forelimb affected by the ulcerated swelling showed an osteolytic lesion of the radius. A fine-needle aspirate was taken from the radial lesion (163) (May–Gruenwald–Giemsa stain).
i. What diagnosis does the cytology support?
ii. What tests can be used to confirm the diagnosis?
iii. What is the diagnostic value of antigen testing?
iv. What treatment should be performed?

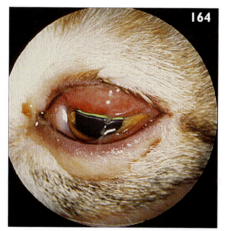

164 A 4-year-old castrated male Persian cat was seen because of a runny eye. On physical examination, there was marked chemosis and blepharospasm of the affected eye (164). A clear, reddish brown discharge was seen below that eye, and there was a dried crust in the medial canthus.
i. What could be the cause of this problem?
ii. What further preliminary diagnostic steps should be taken?

179

163 i. The sample from the radial lesion contains numerous round to oval, narrow-based budding encapsulated yeast organisms, consistent with *Cryptococcus neoformans*. Cryptococcosis should be suspected in case of rhinitis, sinusitis, CNS involvement, and cutaneous or mucosal lesions in the nasal or oral area. Less commonly it can involve bones, eyes, lungs, and other organs. Cutaneous involvement reflects hematogenous dissemination from the primary site of infection. Localized cutaneous cryptococcosis can develop following penetrating injury of the skin. In some cats, the infection spreads to the mandibular lymph nodes from the nasal cavity or through the cribriform plate into the olfactory bulbs and olfactory tract causing meningoencephalitis or optic neuritis and secondary retinitis.

ii. A serum cryptococcal capsular antigen test and culture are the most widely utilized confirmatory tests.

iii. Tests for cryptococcal antigen in serum are highly sensitive (90–100%) and specific (97–100%). However, false-negative results can occur, especially in cases of localized lesions. When performed properly, antigen testing is also useful to document the response to treatment: a decreasing antigen titer indicates a favorable response and a good prognosis, whereas a persistent titer during treatment suggests resistance.

iv. The drugs of choice are itraconazole and fluconazole; the latter is recommended particularly if ocular or CNS disease is present. In refractory cases, amphotericin B may be administered SC, in infusion, two to three times per week and continued until there has been demonstrable clinical improvement and corresponding decline in the serum antigen titer. The cumulative dose of 10–20 mg/kg appears to be important, rather than the period over which the drug is administered (see **44**). Treatment with a triazole antifungal is administered until the antigen test has been negative for at least 1–2 months. Relapses following cessation of drug are common.

164 i. Differential diagnoses include corneal laceration from trauma or foreign body, entropion, *Chlamydophila felis* infection, corneal laceration, and severe anterior uveitis due to numerous causes. FHV infection is less likely due to the unilateral presentation and the lack of concurrent respiratory signs.

ii. Topical anesthesia for a thorough examination of the globe and adnexa is warranted. With analgesia, evaluation of the anterior chamber, iris, pupil, posterior chamber, and retina may be possible. IOPs should be assessed. The unaffected eye should be checked first to minimize the possibility of transmission of infectious agents. Fluorescein stain uptake should be performed to identify any superficial erosions. Conjunctival scrapings can be made for cytologic evaluation looking for inclusion bodies characteristic of *C. felis* infection. *C. felis* inclusion bodies were found in this cat. Treatment with oral doxycycline 10 mg/kg/day for 28 days eliminated the infection. Because doxycycline can cause esophageal stricture formation, each dose must be chased with a 3–6 ml water bolus.

165 A 9-year-old spayed female Persian cat was seen because of a history of chronic vomiting. Complete blood count, serum biochemical panel, urinalysis, blood pressure, and abdominal radiographs were normal. Gastric and intestinal biopsies were collected. On histopathology, there was a tangle of spiral-shaped bacteria within the gastric gland with modest edema and hyperplasia of the gastric

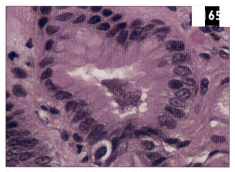

mucosa (165). Scattered lymphocytes, plasma cells, and lymphoid aggregates were seen in the submucosa and lamina propria.
i. What is the significance of spiral-shaped organisms in the gastric biopsy?
ii. What therapy should be recommended?
iii. Is this condition of zoonotic significance?

166 A 10-year-old castrated male domestic shorthair cat was seen because of a sudden change in mentation. It was an indoor-only cat. An FIV antibody test at the age of 5 months had been positive. On presentation, the cat appeared irritable and depressed and the left side of the face was twitching continuously. On clinical examination, the cat reacted painfully when the cervical spine was palpated. It was otherwise unremarkable apart from the neurologic signs.

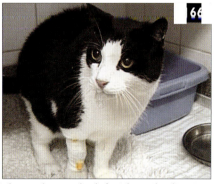

There was continuous twitching of the facial muscles on the left side and salivation (166). The neurologic examination demonstrated decreased menace response of the right eye with normal pupil size and pupillary light reflexes, and delayed hopping of the right pelvic limb. Hematologic and biochemical evaluation showed mild leukopenia, lymphopenia, and hyperproteinemia, with normal albumin but marked hyperglobulimemia.
i. What is the neuroanatomical localization?
ii. What are the differential diagnoses?

165 i. The organisms resemble *Helicobacter* spp. These can be present in gastric biopsies from clinically healthy cats as well as cats with gastrointestinal disease, thus, it is difficult to attribute a pathogenic role to them. They may be commensals, opportunists that participate in illness in predisposed individuals, or causative agents themselves in some individuals.

ii. Therapy for *Helicobacter* spp. infections is controversial in cats because of its questionable role in disease. Treatment regimes are adapted from those used in people and include drugs that increase pH (e.g. omeprazole, famotidine) with two or three antimicrobial agents (e.g. metronidazole, amoxicillin, clarithromycin, doxycycline). The role of the pH-increasing drugs is to make the gastric environment less hospitable for these bacteria.

iii. Most epidemiologic studies do not support an association between cat contact and human *H. pylori* infection. Most cats that have spiral-shaped organisms in their stomachs, healthy or with clinical signs of gastritis, have not had their *Helicobacter* spp. typed. In those that have, *H. pylori* is rare. Thus, while not impossible, feline gastric helicobacteriosis should not be a significant public health concern. In humans, *H. pylori* is associated not only with peptic ulcers, but also with neoplasia. In cats, any association between *Helicobacter* spp. and neoplasia is not clearly established.

166 i. The observed episode of unilateral facial muscle twitching, salivation, and abnormal mental status represents a focal seizure. In this case, the onset of lateralized focal seizures in an older cat suggests structural brain disease. This was also suggested by the visual abnormalities: unilateral menace deficit with a normal pupillary light reflex indicates central blindness (left occipital lobe) or cerebellar disease. Thus, the neurologic presentation is more suggestive of multifocal than focal intracranial disease, because seizures and neurologic deficits appear to arise from different sides of the forebrain.

ii. The primary differential for recent-onset multifocal intracranial disease is CNS inflammation (encephalitis, meningoencephalitis). Neoplasia (lymphoma, meningioma, and other types of neoplasia) must also be considered because of the advanced age of the cat, as well as cerebrovascular accidents (infarcts), because of the sudden onset of neurologic signs. Metabolic or toxic causes are unlikely with lateralized seizures and lateralized neurologic deficits. CNS inflammation is routinely diagnosed by CSF analysis or combined MRI/CSF analysis. Prior to anesthesia for MRI/CSF collection, a complete blood count and biochemistry panel should be performed to detect metabolic or inflammatory diseases. Metastatic neoplasia may be ruled out with thoracic radiographs and abdominal ultrasonography. Neuroimaging, preferably with MRI is usually done prior to CSF analysis within the same anesthetic episode to assess increased intracranial pressure from hydrocephalus or neoplasia.

167 Case 167 is the same cat as case 166. CT imaging of the brain showed patchy contrast enhancement throughout the left cerebral cortex with some mass effect and additional periventricular contrast enhancement. CSF collected under general anesthesia was found to contain an increased leukocyte count (8 cells/µl) but normal protein (0.14 g/l). Differential cell count revealed a mixed pleocytosis with neutrophils, monocytes,

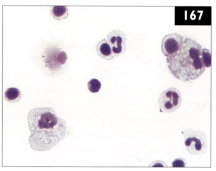

and lymphocytes (167). The serum *Toxoplasma gondii* IgM antibody titer was 1:1024 (high), and IgG antibody titer was 1:512 (moderate). Although the cat had been tested FIV-positive at the age of 5 months, it was now negative for FIV antibodies and FeLV antigen.
i. What is the diagnosis?
ii. How should the cat be treated?
iii. What is the assessment of the different FIV antibody test results?

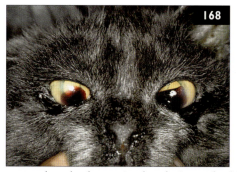

168 A 5-year-old castrated male domestic shorthair cat had been living as an indoor-only cat in a single-cat household for 3 years. The cat was seen because of bleeding in the anterior chamber of the eye (168). The bleeding was caused by a severe thrombocytopenia (35 × 10⁹/l). The cat tested positive for FeLV antigen.
i. Can FeLV infection cause the clinical signs in this cat?
ii. Is antiviral chemotherapy useful in FeLV-infected cats?

167 i. The CSF analysis indicates the presence of CNS inflammation. A mixed cell pattern is typically seen with FIP, protozoal infections, some meningiomas, and resorptive lesions. CT is usually poorly suited to evaluation of the neuroparenchyma, and, therefore, is not very helpful here. Nevertheless, patchy contrast uptake is compatible with CNS inflammation. The high *T. gondii* IgM antibody titer suggests infection with *T. gondii* but does not necessarily imply active disease. Moderate and high IgM antibody titers are also seen in chronic asymptomatic infections. Toxoplasmosis should never be diagnosed with a single elevated IgG or IgM antibody titer. Instead, retesting after 3–4 weeks with demonstration of a fourfold rise or fall in the IgM antibody titer is recommended or demonstration of the organism by PCR. Nevertheless, toxoplasmosis seems to be the most likely diagnosis here.
ii. In this cat, anticonvulsive treatment with phenobarbital was given, along with clindamycin for the treatment of systemic and CNS toxoplasmosis. Alternatively, toxoplasmosis could be treated with sulfonamide/trimethoprim or sulphonamide/pyrimethamine to avoid the side-effects of clindamycin. The cat was healthy and seizure-free 2 years after the initial presentation.
iii. Since FIV causes lifelong infection, it is likely that the positive FIV antibody test at 5 months of age was not caused by infection but by maternal antibodies from a queen that was infected with or vaccinated against FIV. Vaccine is available in the USA, where this cat was born.

168 i. FeLV can cause thrombocytopenia. It can cause either decreased production or immune-mediated destruction of the platelets.
ii. Most antiviral drugs are specifically intended for treatment of human immunodeficiency virus (HIV) infection, but some can be used to treat FeLV infection. All the drugs mentioned below inhibit FeLV replication *in vitro*, but efficacy *in vivo* is limited in most of them. (1) AZT (zidovudine) should only be used at low dosage (5 mg/kg PO or SC q 12 h) in FeLV-infected cats due to its bone marrow-suppressive effects, and cats with pre-existing FeLV-associated bone marrow suppression should not be treated. (2) Zalcitabine, didanosine, ribavirin, foscarnet, and suramin all cause side-effects in cats and are not clinically useful. (3) Human interferon-α has been tried, but it did not result in any statistically significant differences in FeLV status, survival time, clinical or hematologic parameters, or improvement in the owners' subjective impression. (4) Feline interferon-ω was recently licensed for use in veterinary medicine in some European countries and Japan. In one study, a statistically significant difference was noted in the survival time of treated *vs.* untreated cats. No virologic parameters, however, were measured throughout the study to support the hypothesis that interferon actually had an anti-FeLV effect rather than inhibited secondary infections, and further studies are needed.

169 A 2-year-old spayed female domestic shorthair cat was seen for its annual health care visit (169). The cat was an indoor/outdoor cat and lived together with nine other healthy cats. It had received its primary vaccination series (FPV, FHV, FCV) at the age of 8 weeks and 12 weeks and rabies vaccine at 12 weeks, and all vaccines had been given again 1 year later. On physical examination, there was nothing remarkable except a slightly reduced BCS (2/5) and a rough hair coat. However, the cat tested positive on a FeLV antigen test (FIV antibody-negative).

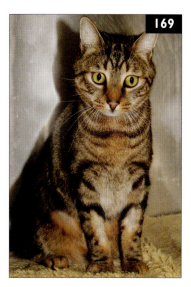

i. What does a positive FeLV antigen test mean?
ii. What is the course of FeLV infection?

170 Case 170 is the same cat as case 169 (170). The cat lived together with nine other cats in the same household.
i. What should be done with the other cats?
ii. How high is the risk of transmission to the other cats?
iii. Should the other cats in that household be vaccinated against FeLV?

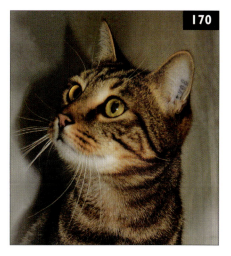

169 i. This may be a false-positive result or the cat may truly be infected. This blood sample was retested with a different test and was positive again. Thus, a false-positive result is very unlikely.

ii. The outcome of FeLV infection varies; it depends on the immune status, the cat's age, the pathogenicity of the virus strain, and the virus concentration. After initial infection, usually *via* the oronasal route, virus replicates in the lymphoid tissue. In many immunocompetent cats, virus replication stops now. Such cats develop strong immunity. If the immune response is inadequate, FeLV spreads within lymphocytes and monocytes, free FeLV p27 antigen is detectable, and cats become positive on plasma antigen tests. These cats may shed virus. Often, viremia ends within 3–6 weeks. After about 3 weeks, hematopoietic precursor cells in the bone marrow become infected, releasing infected granulocytes and platelets. After this, intracellular antigen is also detectable. Cats cannot now completely eliminate the virus even if they do not remain viremic, as its DNA is integrated into the bone marrow cells. These cats are negative on routine tests for FeLV antigen. However, infection can be reactivated spontaneously or after immunosuppression, and cats can become viremic again. If initial viremia persists for longer than 16 weeks, the cat becomes persistently viremic ('progressive infection'), and may develop FeLV-associated diseases; most of these die within 3 years.

170 i. All cats should be tested to determine their FeLV status. If one or more positive cats are identified, the owner must be informed that the best method of preventing spread to others is to isolate the infected individuals. In this case, all nine other cats tested negative for FeLV.

ii. The risk of transmission is not very high in such a situation. If one FeLV-infected cat has been living in an otherwise negative household, the other cats will have been infected by the FeLV-shedding cat and are probably immune by now. However, a previously immune cat may become viremic, due either to new infection or to reactivation of a long-persisting latent infection. If an owner elects to keep them all, the risk of infection is approximately 10–15% for an adult cat if it lives with a viremic cat for months or years.

iii. If owners refuse to separate housemates, the uninfected cats should be vaccinated to enhance their natural level of immunity. However, owners should realize that vaccination does not provide high levels of protection in such a highly infectious situation. No new FeLV-negative cats should be introduced into the household, as vaccination will not protect them sufficiently. If the household is closed to new cats, the FeLV-negative cats tend to outlive the progressively infected cats, so that after some time all remaining cats will be immune.

171 An apparently healthy stray young adult intact male domestic shorthair cat was rescued and seen for its first preventive care examination (**171**). Physical examination was normal. Tests for FeLV and FIV were performed, and the FIV antibody test was positive. A PCR submitted for confirmation of FIV infection was, however, negative.

i. What is the interpretation of these test results?

ii. What is the recommendation for this cat based on the FIV test findings?

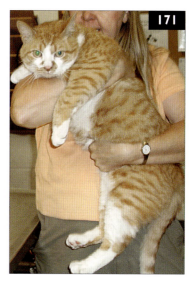

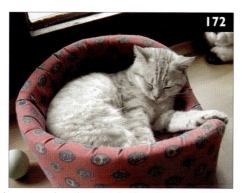

172 A 9-month-old castrated male British Shorthair cat (**172**) was seen because of fever and thoracic effusion. FIP was diagnosed on the basis of immunofluorescence staining of FCoV antigen in macrophages of the effusion. The cat had lived indoors since it was obtained by the owners. It was born in a multi-cat household (18 cats) in northern Germany and was purchased by the owners at the age of 10 weeks.

i. What is the pathogenesis of FIP?

ii. What are risk factors for the development of FIP?

iii. How did the cat become infected?

171 i. An FIV vaccine is available in the USA. Thus, a positive FIV antibody test is consistent with FIV infection, vaccination (or both), or the presence of maternal antibodies (in a cat of less than 6 months of age). In some cats, antibodies induced by FIV vaccination have been observed to persist for at least 5 years after the last vaccine was administered. Currently available tests are unable to distinguish between antibodies induced by infection or vaccination. A negative PCR test indicates the cat either is free of infection or is infected with a strain of FIV having sufficient genetic sequence divergence that the PCR test yields a false-negative result. False-negative results have been reported to occur in 25–50% of cats naturally infected with FIV. Because the cat's vaccination history is unknown, it is not possible to know the cat's true FIV infection status.
ii. Since the cat may be infected, it is recommended that it be neutered and kept in a single-cat indoor home. FIV-infected cats generally have a long (many years) period of good health. Twice annual physical examinations and annual blood count, biochemistry panel, and urinalysis are recommended for early detection and treatment of any abnormalities.

172 i. FIP is caused by a virus FCoV variant that develops within a cat infected with harmless FCoV. FIP develops when there is a spontaneous mutation in the FCoV genome. This leads to changes in the surface structures of the virus, allowing virus binding to ribosomes in macrophages. This mutated virus, in contrast to its harmless relative, becomes able to replicate within macrophages; this is the key event in the pathogenesis of FIP. The disease itself is caused by an immune-mediated reaction to the systemic infection. Within 2 weeks, mutated pathogenic FCoV have been distributed to the cecum, colon, intestinal lymph nodes, spleen, liver, and CNS. FIP occurs as a result of the development of vasculitis and granulomatous changes. The vasculitis leads to DIC.
ii. Immunosuppression may allow for increased intestinal virus replication, making it more likely that a 'virulent mutation' will occur. Many factors increase the probability of the mutation occurring, including young age, breed predisposition, immunosuppression, infection with FeLV or FIV, stress, glucocorticoid treatment, and surgery. Dosage, virulence of the virus strain, and reinfection rate also affect the rate of replication.
iii. Cats are usually infected *via* the oronasal route through contaminated feces shed by cats with harmless FCoV enteric infections. Indirect transmission is also possible, e.g. through clothes, toys, and grooming tools. In this cat, transmission probably occurred before the cat came into the new household.

173 Case 173 is the same cat as case 172. The owner wanted to treat the cat (173). There was a second cat in the household, a 3-year-old neutered female British shorthair cat.

i. What is the prognosis for a cat with FIP?
ii. What are the treatment options?
iii. How high is the risk that FIP will be transmitted to the second cat in the household?

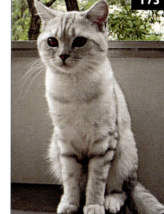

174 An adult (unknown age) female (unknown neutering status) domestic shorthair cat was seen because of fever and dyspnea. It had been found 7 days earlier in the middle of a city. On physical examination, the cat showed fever (body temperature 40.5°C), lethargy, emaciation, dehydration, tachypnea, dyspnea, and had increased bronchial lung sounds. Thoracic radiographs revealed an interstitial and alveolar pattern with partial consolidation and emphysema (174a). The cat was euthanized due to rapid deterioration. Necropsy findings consisted of disseminated nodular infiltrations of the lungs and mediastinal lymph nodes. Histopathology of these organs revealed a granulomatous inflammation with a large number of acid-fast bacteria (174b). Molecular biology tests demonstrated the presence of nucleic acid sequences consistent with *Mycobacterium tuberculosis*.

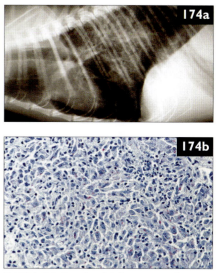

i. How common is *M. tuberculosis* in cats?
ii. What are the typical clinical signs?
iii. Should infected cats be treated?

173 i. After a definitive diagnosis of FIP, the prognosis is very poor. In a recent study, the median survival time after definitive diagnosis was 8 days. However, there is much individual variation; survival times of 6 months and longer have been reported.

ii. As FIP is an immune-mediated disease, treatment is aimed at controlling the immune response to FcoV. Immunosuppressive drugs such as prednisolone (2–4 mg/kg PO q 24 h) or cyclophosphamide (2 mg/kg PO q 48 h) may slow disease progression but will not cure FIP. Feline interferon-ω has been used, but was not effective in a placebo-controlled study. This cat was treated with prednisolone and feline interferon-ω. The effusion resolved, and the cat was clinically healthy for 6 months. Then it developed upper respiratory tract disease and uveitis. During the next 3 weeks, its general condition deteriorated, and the cat was euthanized 200 days after treatment initiation. At necropsy, FIP was reconfirmed.

iii. Transmission of the mutated FIP-causing FCoV is very unlikely under natural circumstances. Therefore, there is no increased risk for the second cat in the household, which is probably already infected with the harmless FCoV.

174 i. *M. tuberculosis* infection is extremely rare in cats (much rarer than in dogs). Tuberculosis is caused by *M. tuberculosis* and *M. bovis*, which both require infection of reservoir mammalian hosts, because environmental survival is limited to a maximum of 2 weeks. Humans are the only reservoir hosts of *M. tuberculosis*; if cats are infected, it is through contact with infected humans. *M. bovis* is closely related to *M. tuberculosis* and is difficult to distinguish from it, except by biochemical tests and nucleic acid probes. *M. bovis*, too, does not exist long in the environment, and reservoir hosts are essential.

ii. Infection with *M. tuberculosis* in cats (and dogs) is often asymptomatic or insidious. *M. tuberculosis* has an affinity for tissues with high oxygen content, and this explains its common localization in the lungs. In pulmonary manifestations, bronchopneumonia, pulmonary nodule formation, and hilar lymphadenopathy are seen, causing fever, weight loss, anorexia, and harsh, nonproductive coughing. Animals with tuberculous pneumonitis discharge organisms in the sputum, and aerosolized droplets are the primary means of transmission.

iii. Although pets acquire *M. tuberculosis* infection from people, and the spread from cats (or dogs) to people has not been reported, infected animals are a potential risk to humans and euthanasia should be considered.

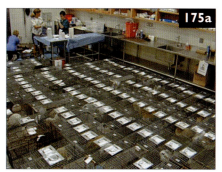

175 In some countries (e.g. the USA), large-scale feral cat neutering programs frequently trap and perform surgery on more than 100 cats in a day (175a). Due to the wild nature of undomesticated feral cats they may be handled safely only under anesthesia, and they are unlikely to be retrapped to receive additional veterinary care in the future.

i. What is the ideal vaccination program in this situation?

ii. Should feral cats in trap–neuter–return (TNR) programs be tested for FeLV or FIV?

iii. How should these vaccinated cats be marked for identification?

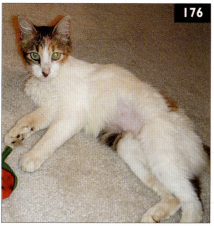

176 An 8-year-old spayed female domestic longhair cat was referred for examination because of recurrent fever and lethargy of 4 months' duration (176). The cat lived exclusively indoors with another cat, which was healthy. On physical examination, body temperature was increased (39.8°C), the cat had poor BCS (score 3/9) and haircoat, and there was generalized peripheral lympha-denopathy. Previous treatment with appropriate dosages of amoxicillin, enrofloxacin, and azithromycin had not resolved the fever. Tests for FeLV and FIV were negative.

i. What are the three major etiologic categories of fever?

ii. What is the best approach for diagnosing the cause of fever of unknown origin (FUO) in this cat?

175 i. Despite the stressful experiences of trapping, transportation, anesthesia, and surgery, adult feral cats have been shown to respond well to vaccination performed under anesthesia at the time of surgery. Ideally, feral cats would be vaccinated against FPV, FHV, and FCV when they are handled for surgery. Public health concerns dictate that all cats be immunized against rabies in endemic areas. Since the efficacy of a single FeLV vaccination is unknown and adds considerable costs to neutering programs, it is not usually included. Vaccination not

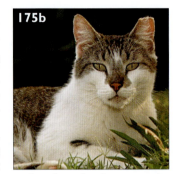

175b

only protects the individual feral cat receiving the vaccine, but also improves the disease resistance and health of the colony to which it is returned.

ii. The prevalence of FeLV and FIV infection in feral cat colonies tends to mirror the low values of housecats that venture outdoors. For this reason and because neutering reduces the highest risk factors for viral transmission (reproduction and fighting), many large-scale feral cat neutering programs do not invest resources in testing.

iii. Feral cats participating in TNR programs should have an ear tipped for identification (175b).

176 i. The most common causes of fever are: (1) infectious inflammation, (2) non-infectious inflammation (e.g. autoimmune diseases), and (3) neoplasia.

ii. Diagnosis of the cause of FUO is often a protracted and frustrating process. The plan should include a logical series of diagnostic steps to rule out the most common causes of fever first, and then to consider uncommon causes. Initial tests should be minimally invasive and proceed to more invasive procedures if preliminary tests are nondiagnostic. A complete blood count, biochemical panel, and urinalysis should be performed. In this case, there was generalized lymphadenopathy, so fine-needle aspirates of the lymph nodes are included as part of the initial evaluation. If the cause is not identified upon the initial testing, ANA, thoracic and abdominal radiographs, and abdominal ultrasonography with fine-needle aspirates of any abnormalities should also be performed. If a diagnosis still is not apparent, further evaluation should include blood and urine cultures, joint fluid and CSF analysis, cardiac ultrasonography to rule out endocarditis, and tests for the regionally prevalent viral, bacterial, rickettsial, fungal, and protozoal pathogens.

177 Case 177 is the same cat as case 176. Complete blood count, biochemistry panel, and urinalysis were performed. Cytologic evaluation of the lymph node aspirate revealed a mixed population of small and large lymphocytes with an increased number of plasma cells. No organisms or neoplastic cells were seen (177). Cytologic evaluation of joint fluid revealed an increased

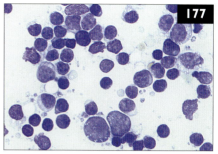

number of nondegenerate neutrophils. Protein electrophoresis indicated a polyclonal gammopathy and the ANA titer was 1:128. Blood and urine cultures were negative. Radiography of the thorax and abdomen and ultrasonography of the abdomen and heart were normal. The owner declined CSF collection.

Blood profile/ biochemistry panel	Results	Blood profile/ biochemistry panel	Results
Hematocrit	0.26 l/l	Albumin	23 g/l
RBC	4.5×10^{12}/l	Globulins	61 g/l
Hemoglobin	5.0 mmol/l	**Urinalysis** (cystocentesis)	
WBC	19.5×10^9/l	Protein	++++
Mature neutrophils	17.5×10^9/l	Protein : creatinine	3.5
Lymphocytes	1.0×10^9/l	Specific gravity	1.045
Total protein	84 g/l	Color/appearance	yellow, hazy

i. What do the cytologic findings in the lymph node and joint fluid indicate?
ii. What is the interpretation of the laboratory values?
iii. What is the diagnosis?
iv. What is the treatment plan?
v. What is the prognosis?

178 A 6-year-old spayed female domestic shorthair cat was seen for routine annual examination and consultation. The owner did not have any concerns about its health. On physical examination both plaque and calculus were present on the teeth, and there was gingival recession at several roots. The gingiva was noted to be especially inflamed at these sites (178), and halitosis was noted.

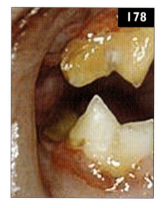

i. What is the condition seen in this cat?
ii. How do plaque and calculus differ and why are they important?
iii. What is the most common organism causing periodontitis?

177 i. The lymph node is reactive and the joint fluid indicates active inflammation.
ii. There is a mild nonregenerative anemia, suggesting anemia of chronic inflammation, and a stress leukogram, a common response to inflammation in cats. Mild hyperglobulinemia and hypoalbuminemia are present; protein electrophoresis confirms a polyclonal gammopathy consistent with a chronic inflammatory response. Proteinuria in the absence of an inflammatory urine sediment or microbial growth suggests an immune-mediated glomerulopathy. The positive ANA test suggests systemic lupus erythematosus (SLE).
iii. The tentative diagnosis is SLE. This can involve multiple organ systems and is frequently associated with peripheral lymphadenopathy in cats. There is often a history of antibiotic-unresponsive fever as well. Immune-mediated diseases are frequently diagnosed after eliminating infectious or neoplastic conditions.

This case illustrates that the presence of fever and leukocytosis does not always indicate the presence of infection.
iv. In this case, treatment was started with prednisolone, after which the lymphadenopathy resolved. Lethargy and recurrent fever persisted, so chlorambucil was added. The cat went into complete remission, but signs relapsed following attempts to reduce the medication. SLE is a chronic condition; treatment is aimed at controlling the inflammatory response while minimizing drug side-effects. If the diagnosis is incorrect or a concurrent infectious disease is present, therapy may promote dissemination of the infection.
v. The prognosis of feline SLE is fair to good if an initial remission is easily induced. Many cats eventually become resistant to treatment or develop organ failure as a result of the inflammatory process.

178 i. Periodontal disease may be described as inflammation and recession of perialveolar gingival margins. It is extremely common in cats and is initiated by the presence of plaque. This biofilm is created by normal resident microflora as a by-product of food breakdown and saliva. It acts as an organic matrix of salivary glycoproteins and polysaccharides adhering to enamel and providing sites for bacteria to proliferate.
ii. Calculus is the mineralized form of plaque. It facilitates further formation of plaque as well as periodontal inflammation. Thus both supra- and subgingival calculus and plaque must be thoroughly removed in order to control periodontal disease.
iii. *Porphyromonas (Bacteriodes) gingivalis* is associated with the progression of periodontal disease in cats.

179 Case 179 is the same cat as case 178. Radiographs of the teeth were taken (179).

i. What role do antimicrobials play in the treatment of this condition?

ii. Regarding the tooth shown in the radiograph, what treatment should be recommended?

iii. What systemic complications of periodontal disease may occur?

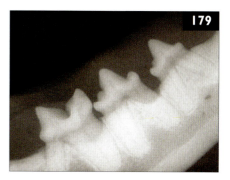

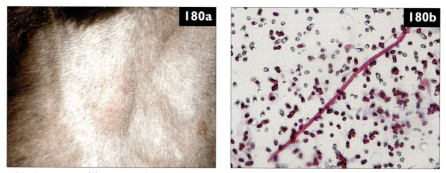

180 A 2-year-old neutered male domestic shorthair cat was seen because of a 3-month history of cutaneous nodules on the left side of the thorax and the neck (180a). It was an indoor/outdoor cat living in Florence, Italy. On physical examination, the cat was alert and responsive, but very thin. Thoracic auscultation was unremarkable. There were well-circumscribed nonpainful subcutaneous nodules (1 cm in diameter) on the neck and thorax. Initial evaluation consisted of a complete blood count, biochemistry panel, urinalysis, and FeLV and FIV tests. Cytology of the skin nodules was also performed. Complete blood count revealed eosinophilia. FeLV antigen and FIV antibody tests were negative. On the blood smear, a single microfilaria of *Dirofilaria immitis* was detected (180b).

i. What differential diagnoses should be considered?

ii. What is the plan to confirm the diagnosis?

iii. What is the frequency of microfilaremia in heartworm disease in cats?

179 i. Antimicrobials are a component of periodontal therapy, but without conscientious dental prophylaxis, progression of periodontal disease is likely to continue. Appropriate antibiotics are clindamycin, doxycycline, or spiramycin combined with metronidazole. Amoxicillin/clavulanate, despite sensitivity profiles, does not decrease the numbers of *Porphyromonas gingivalis*.
ii. In addition to mechanical scaling and antimicrobial therapy, severely affected teeth should be extracted. Debridement of the adjacent necrotic tissue and proliferative gingival margins should also be undertaken.
iii. In people, cerebral and myocardial infarction may occur; in dogs, cardiac, renal, and hepatic disease may follow. In cats (and dogs), there may be ophthalmic complications from periodontal inflammation and infection of the caudal maxillary teeth. These include pain on opening the mouth with resultant anorexia, fever, chemosis, conjunctival hyperemia, exophthalmoses, and protrusion of the third eyelid.

180 i. Nodular subcutaneous lesions are usually inflammatory or neoplastic; noninflammatory benign lesions are uncommon. Foreign-body reactions and parasitic granulomas are other possibilities. In this case cytologic examination of samples obtained by fine-needle aspiration revealed degenerate neutrophils and macrophages, with some plasma cells and histiocytes. These findings were consistent with pyogranulomatous inflammation. A lesion that contains both non-degenerate neutrophils and a prominent fraction of mononuclear phagocytes indicates a more chronic response and fungi, bacteria (e.g. actinomycosis, nocardiosis, mycobacteriosis), and protozoa must be considered.

The finding of a dirofilarial microfilaria in the circulation indicates a patent heartworm infection in this cat. On the basis of the cytology result, a biopsy for histopathology was performed.
ii. Additional tests include antibody and antigen tests for *D. immitis* and staining for acid-fast or fungal organisms in tissue biopsies. Interpretation of heartworm tests may be complicated for many reasons. However, the sensitivity of commercially available tests has increased, and now they are highly effective in detecting single adult female worm infestations. In the cat, detectable antigenemia develops at about 5–8 months postinfection. Thus, the clinical signs of heartworm infection may be present prior to the presence of detectable antigenemia.
iii. In the vast majority of cases of feline heartworm disease, cats are amicrofilaremic. If they are present, microfilariae are usually those of *D. immitis* (**180c**), but in northern Italy, microfilariae of *D. repens* have also been found.

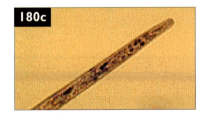

180c

181 Case 181 is the same cat as case 180. The heartworm antibody test was positive in this cat. Cytology of the fine-needle aspirates showed pyogranulomatous inflammation with degenerate neutrophils and macrophages. A complete surgical resection of one of the nodules was performed. Histology shows a section of a *Dirofilaria immitis* microfilaria within a nodule of pyogranulomatous inflammation (181).

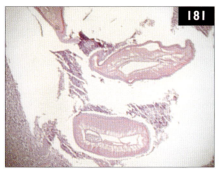

i. What are the clinical signs and what is the outcome in cats with heartworm disease?
ii. What are typical findings in diagnostic imaging?

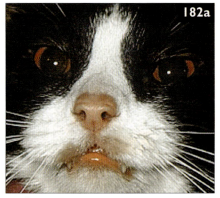

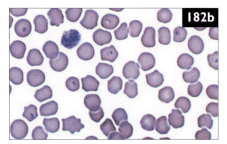

182 A 5-year-old castrated male domestic shorthair cat was seen in the USA because of a 3-day history of progressive depression. It was allowed indoors and outdoors. It was current on vaccinations. The cat had had negative FeLV and FIV tests the previous year. On physical examination, the cat was depressed and icteric (182a). There was fever (body temperature 39.8°C), tachycardia (200 bpm), and tachypnea (50 bpm). Complete blood count, biochemical panel, clotting profile, and urinalysis revealed nonregenerative anemia, leukopenia, thrombocytopenia, increased ALT activity and ALP activity, hyperbilirubinemia, hyperammonemia, increased PTT, and increased FDPs. On examination of the blood smear, intraerythocytic piroplasms with 'safety pin' morphology were observed in a few cells (182b).
i. What is the diagnosis?
ii. What is the treatment for this disease?
iii. What is the prognosis?

181 i. In cats, *D. immitis* infection and consequent heartworm disease are quite common in endemic areas, but the infection rate is only 5–20% of that of dogs. Worm burdens are usually low (1–2 worms) but morbidity and mortality tend to be greater than in dogs. A small worm burden can cause sudden death, chronic vomiting, coughing, dyspnea, respiratory failure, and weight loss. Many other symptoms may be seen, including tachycardia, syncope, and central nervous system abnormalities. Often, the clinical signs may be confused with signs of bronchial asthma. Skin lesions due to microfilaria or adult worms are rare; infrequently, *D. immitis* larvae or adults may result in the formation of nodular to ulcerative lesions or a papular pruritic rash due to a hypersensitivity reaction to larvae. Aberrant adult heartworms have been recovered from many sites and the most reported cases are incidental findings.

ii. As in dogs, radiography and echocardiography are useful in cats. Thoracic radiography may provide strong evidence of feline heartworm disease, and is valuable for assessing the severity of disease and monitoring its progression or regression. On echocardiography, heartworms are seen as a double-lined echodensity in about 50% of cats diagnosed with heartworm infection. In some cases, worms are not visualized. Cardiac ultrasound examination and thoracic radiographs did not show any findings associated with dirofilariasis in this case.

182 i. The diagnosis is *Cytauxzoon felis* infection, a tick-borne protozoal infection of domestic and nondomestic cats. The infection is usually asymptomatic in the reservoir host (bobcat) and other nondomestic felids. In domestic cats, infection typically results in a rapidly progressive course of hemolytic anemia, respiratory and hepatic failure, DIC, and shock. The time from the first clinical signs to death is often approximately 5 days.

ii. Treatment consists of supportive care and antiprotozoal treatment. Numerous drugs have been tried with variable success. Recently, combination therapy with atovaquone and azithromycin has been used and may prove superior to other drugs.

iii. Cats that present in the later stages of disease with hypothermia, DIC, and coma have a poor prognosis for survival. Cats that survive the first 3 days of therapy have a favorable prognosis. Recently, a higher survival rate, even among untreated cats, has been reported, suggesting that less virulent strains or host adaptation are developing. Nonetheless, this cat died before treatment could be initiated.

183 A 14-year-old castrated male domestic shorthair cat was seen because of coughing. It was allowed to roam outside. Six months earlier, the cat had been diagnosed with pulmonary cryptococcosis and FIV infection. The cat had been treated with oral itraconazole for the past 6 months. The cough had resolved. Its serum cryptococcal antigen titer had declined from a pretreatment value of 1:256 to zero. The cryptococcal antigen test was repeated when the cough recurred, and was still negative. Thoracic radiographs showed a diffuse bronchointerstitial pattern. A BAL was performed and on cytology, mainly macrophages, a few eosinophils, and a few neutrophils were seen. Three large nematodes were seen in the bronchial wash fluid (183) (wet preparation).

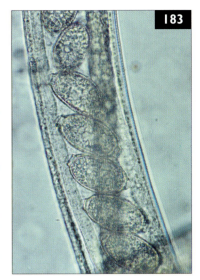

i. What nematode species is this?
ii. How should the cat be treated?
iii. What is the significance of the cat's FIV status?

184 An outbreak of upper respiratory tract disease characterized by oral and corneal ulceration, conjunctivitis, fever, nasal discharge, and sneezing occurred in multiple rooms at a cat rescue facility. All cats had been tested negative for FeLV and FIV at the time of admission and had received MLV vaccines against FPV, FHV, and FCV at admission and

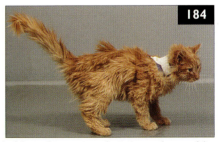

3 weeks later. Parasite control was provided by selemectin administered monthly. Cats remained in their originally assigned room from the time of admission to the time of adoption. Of the 120 cats kept in the facility, the most severely affected were kittens aged 8 weeks to 4 months. One litter of 4-month-old kittens that had resided at the facility for 5 weeks was particularly ill, with severe oral ulceration, salivation, anorexia, fever, and dehydration (184).

i. What are the differential diagnoses?
ii. What is the treatment?
iii. Is the preventive health care program appropriate?

183 i. Within the body of the female nematode are several trichurid, double operculated ova with asymmetric bipolar plugs characteristic of *Eucoleus aerophila* (formerly *Capillaria aerophila*).

ii. Specific treatment protocols have not been evaluated in cats, but fenbendazole and ivermectin have been used successfully. A fecal flotation should be performed post-treatment to ensure elimination of infection.

iii. It is likely that FIV infection with immune dysfunction manifested clinically as sequential respiratory infections. In healthy adult cats, *Eucoleus aerophila* infections are usually asymptomatic. Quantification of lymphocyte subsets (e.g. CD4$^+$ cells, CD8$^+$ cells) or viral load may help clarify whether the cat had immunosuppression associated with chronic FIV infection. However, lymphocyte subset numbers may not be useful as a marker of immune dysfunction in FIV-infected cats since impaired lymphocyte responsiveness precedes the decline in CD4$^+$ cell counts, and some chronically infected cats have very low CD4$^+$ cell counts without obvious clinical immunodeficiency.

184 i. The clinical signs suggest an outbreak of viral upper respiratory tract infection. The combination of both severe ocular and oral lesions suggests a mixed infection with FHV and FCV, but this cannot be confirmed without virus isolation. The other common cause of upper respiratory tract disease in cats is *Bordetella bronchiseptica*. Although it does not typically cause corneal and oral ulceration, it can be present in mixed infections.

ii. In acute infections, treatment is symptomatic while the infection runs its course over several weeks. Antibiotics are used to treat secondary bacterial infections. In group outbreaks, antibiotics should be selected with activity against *B. bronchiseptica* and that can be administered once daily, for practicality. L-lysine supplementation has been suggested in the past, but has been shown to be ineffective or possibly harmful in shelter situations. Topical antibiotic ointment should be applied if there is conjunctivitis or corneal ulceration. Oral famciclovir may be indicated in some cats with FHV infection. The most severely affected cats may need esophagostomy tubes to maintain hydration and nutrition.

iii. The preventive health program, which includes FeLV and FIV testing, MLV vaccination at admission, and routine parasite control, is appropriate. In shelters, vaccinations may be repeated at 2-week intervals until kittens are at least 16 weeks old. Adult cats should be vaccinated twice. Ideally, a quarantine area would be available to house newly arriving cats. FHV and FCV are highly infectious and can be easily transmitted by contaminated equipment or personnel, so thorough cleaning with appropriate cleaning solutions is required. Many routinely used disinfectants, such as quaternary ammonium products, do not inactivate both viruses.

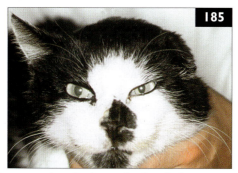

185 A 15-year-old castrated male domestic shorthair cat was seen for its annual health check. The cat had been tested FIV-positive 8 years ago. At the time of diagnosis the cat was an intact male, mainly outdoor cat that used to fight. It had lost one ear in a conflict with the neighbors' dog (185). Since the diagnosis of the FIV infection, the cat had been neutered and became a single indoor-only cat. It occasionally suffered from mild ocular and nasal discharge and stomatitis, but was otherwise healthy.

i. What is the prognosis in FIV infection?
ii. How should a FIV-infected cat be managed at home?
iii. Should a FIV-infected cat receive routine vaccinations?

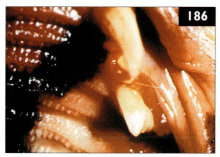

186 Case 186 is the same cat as case 185. On physical examination, the cat had some ocular discharge on the left side and slightly protruding third eyelids on both sides. It also had gingivitis around some of its teeth (186).

i. How often should FIV-infected cats receive health-check visits to their veterinarian?
ii. What has to be considered if FIV-infected cats need veterinary care?
iii. What has to be considered if FIV-infected cats are sick?

185 i. FIV can cause an acquired immunodeficiency syndrome in cats resulting in an increased risk of opportunistic infections, neurologic diseases, and tumors. In most naturally infected cats, however, FIV infection does not cause a severe clinical syndrome. Infected cats can live for many years and may die in old age from causes unrelated to their FIV infection; their quality of life is usually fairly good.

ii. The most important life-prolonging advice is to keep FIV-infected cats strictly indoors. This is not only to prevent spread to other cats in the neighborhood, but also to prevent exposure of the immunosuppressed cat to infectious agents carried by other animals or in the environment. Secondary infections play a major role in the progression of FIV infection. FIV-infected cats should be fed a well-cooked, high-quality diet to avoid the risk of acquiring food-borne bacterial or parasitic infections, and should be neutered to reduce stresses associated with estrus, mating, fighting and the desire to roam outside.

iii. Opinions about vaccination of FIV-infected cats differ. FIV-infected cats are more susceptible to secondary infections; thus, routine vaccination seems to be indicated. However, although vaccination may give protection from infection, it may also cause progression of FIV infection due to immune stimulation causing increased virus production. If infected cats are kept strictly indoors, the risk of being infected may be lower than the possible harmful effect of vaccination.

186 i. Healh-check visits to the veterinarian should be performed at least 6 monthly in order to detect changes in the health status promptly. A complete blood count, biochemistry panel, and urinalysis should be performed annually. If there are changes, laboratory values should be monitored more frequently.

ii. As the virus lives only for seconds outside the host and is susceptible to all disinfectants, routine cleaning procedures will prevent transmission. In a veterinary hospital, FIV-infected cats can be housed (in individual cages) in the same ward as other hospitalized patients. However, they may be immunosuppressed and should be kept away from cats with other infectious diseases. Hospital staff should wash their hands between patients and after handling animals and cleaning cages (primarily to protect the FIV-infected immunosuppressed cat).

iii. If FIV-infected cats are sick, prompt and accurate identification of the secondary disease is essential to allow early therapeutic intervention and a successful outcome. Many cats with FIV infection respond as well as uninfected cats to appropriate medications, although a longer or more aggressive course of therapy may be needed. Corticosteroids and other immunosuppressive or myelosuppressive drugs should only be considered where their use is essential. Griseofulvin has been shown to cause myelosuppression in FIV-infected cats and should not be used. Surgery is generally well tolerated, although perioperative antibiotic administration should be used for all surgeries and dental procedures.

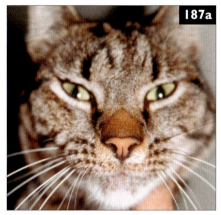

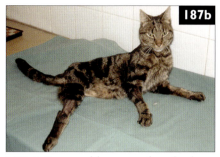

187 A 2-year-old neutered male domestic shorthair cat was referred because of a hind limb injury and progressive neurologic deterioration. It lived mainly outdoors. It had originally been treated by a local veterinarian who had amputated the injured leg. But progressive neurologic signs had developed and the amputation wound had broken down 6 days later. On referral, physical examination showed the cat was in poor body condition and had an unusual facial expression (187a) and moderately increased muscle tone in all three remaining limbs (187b). The cat was hospitalized and the amputation wound was cleaned, debrided, and restitched. When it was offered food the following day, it had a good appetite but was unable to swallow properly. Soon, it was noticed that physical stimulation caused an obvious increase in muscle tone of the remaining limbs.

i. What is the diagnosis?
ii. How should this cat be treated?

188 A 2-year-old spayed female domestic shorthair cat was seen because of recurrent diarrhea (188). The cat was a single, indoor-only cat. Treatment with metronidazole, tylosin, as well as trials with a high-fiber diet, and a low-residue diet had not resolved the diarrhea. Small volumes of cow-pie to semi-formed,

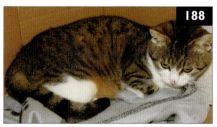

malodorous stool were produced frequently, and intermittently contained mucus and fresh blood. On physical examination, the cat was in good body condition but had a small amount of liquid feces dripping from the anus. Fecal flotation had been negative on two occasions.

i. What portion of the bowel is the problem localized to?
ii. What diagnostic tests should be considered?
iii. How do *Tritrichomonas foetus* and *Giardia lambia* differ microscopically?

187 i. The cat has generalized tetanus. This disease develops as a result of anaerobic infection with *Clostridium tetani* of a wound. *C. tetani* releases an exotoxin (tetanospasmin) which causes inhibition of inhibitory neurotransmitter (GABA, glycine) release in the CNS. This results in uncontrolled contraction of skeletal muscles. The cat's peculiar facial expression, with overly erect ears, narrow palpebral fissures, elevated whiskers, and partial third eyelid prolapse resulted from tetanic contraction of the muscles of facial expression, while dysphagia resulted from pharyngeal muscle spasm. Surprisingly, jaw tone was not increased. The severity of the cat's neurologic signs depended on its state of arousal, with external stimulation resulting in increased muscle tone in the limbs and face. However, cats are relatively resistant to tetanospasmin, so local tetanus is the most common clinical manifestation of tetanus in this species.

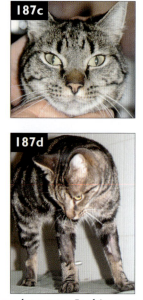

ii. Management of generalized tetanus includes treatment of the inciting wound, neutralization of unbound tetanus toxin in the bloodstream and peripheral tissues using equine antitoxin, and symptomatic therapy to minimize muscle spasm. In this case, the most likely site of clostridial infection was the amputation stump. Accordingly, this wound was debrided and the cat was treated with metronidazole. It improved slowly over 2 weeks, after which time it was essentially normal in its facial expression (187c), and stiffness was no longer present (187d). Feeding these cats can be difficult because of pharyngeal muscle spasm, and insertion of a feeding tube can greatly simplify subsequent management.

188 i. This is large-bowel diarrhea (small amounts, increased frequency, good body condition, mucus, fresh blood). Small-bowel involvement would be associated with normal frequency, variable volume (normal to increased), weight loss, steatorrhea, and melena.
ii. Rectal cytology or direct fecal smear using freshly voided, diarrheic feces diluted with saline and observed under a cover slip may reveal trichomonad trophozoites in approximately 14% of cats infected with *T. foetus*. Culture using commercial kits is simple; in addition, they have a much higher sensitivity. Feces may also be sent to a commercial laboratory with microbiology facilities to be incubated in modified Diamond's medium or for PCR.
iii. *G. lambia* trophozoites have two nuclei, a concave ventral disk and move like a falling leaf. *T. foetus* are spindle-shaped, possess a single nucleus and have an undulating membrane along the entire length of their body. Their movement is jerky and rolling.

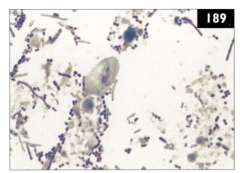

189 Case **189** is the same cat as case **188**. *Tritrichomonas foetus* was identified in the feces of this cat (**189**).
i. How do cats become infected with *T. foetus*?
ii. What are the therapeutic options?
iii. What is the prognosis for a treated *vs*. an untreated cat?

190 A 6-year-old spayed female domestic shorthair cat was seen because of a change of behavior over the past 2 days. It had become apprehensive and nervous, whereas it was normally very friendly. It began seeking solitude and became irritable when approached, even trying to bite people. The cat lived indoors and outdoors in a rural area. It had never been vaccinated. On physical examination the pupils were dilated, and the

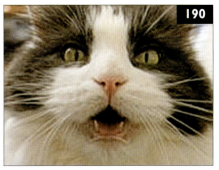

palpebral and corneal reflexes were sluggish. The cat had fever (body temperature 39.9°C) and a blank staring expression. Over the subsequent day in the veterinary hospital, muscle tremors and weakness developed, the cat began to pace in the cage, and further cranial nerve signs developed. It also vocalized frequently, and its voice changed (**190**).
i. What disease should be considered?
ii. What progression of clinical signs is expected?
iii. How is the disease diagnosed?
iv. What therapy is recommended?

189 i. The sources of infection with *T. foetus* are unclear. Numerous potential risk factors have been evaluated. Proximity to pigs, cattle, or horses, type of water source, rural *vs.* urban, recent travel, feeding of raw meat, and outdoor access are not identified as risk factors. Catteries and rescue shelters have a higher prevalence of infection suggesting that hygiene, stress, and other effects of crowding might play a role. It is also possible for a single, indoor-living cat to be infected with *T. foetus*.
ii. Treatment with ronidazole (30 mg/kg q 24 h for 14 days) is effective. This dose should not be exceeded as neurotoxicity may occur. Also, this drug should not be used indiscriminately for diarrhea not confirmed to be due to *T. foetus* due to neurotoxicity that may occur at recommended doses. Not enough is understood at the present time about the pharmacokinetics of this drug in the cat. Many other antimicrobial therapies have been tried unsuccessfully.
iii. In cats treated with ronidazole, long-term cure may be expected. Cats treated with other drugs or untreated can be expected to have recurrent large bowel diarrhea for 4–24 months (median 9 months) before spontaneous resolution of infection occurs.

190 i. Rabies should be considered.
ii. Cats usually develop the furious form of rabies. Paralysis develops rapidly once clinical signs appear.
iii. The diagnosis of rabies is made by the postmortem demonstration of rabies virus antigen in brain tissue. There is no adequately sensitive antemortem test available. Determination of antibodies against rabies virus in blood to document recent exposure to the virus cannot differentiate between antibodies induced by vaccination as compared to infection. Antibody detection is also not reliable as false-negative results may occur.
iv. Treatment of suspected rabies-infected patients is not recommended because no known therapy has proven effective. The risk to the care providers is high, and treatment is not permitted in most countries. Asymptomatic cats suspected of having been exposed to rabies should be reported to local public health authorities, who will decide according to the local laws and vaccination status of the cat and recommend further action (e.g. quarantine, euthanasia). In this case, the cat died suddenly. Histologic evaluation of the brain for Negri bodies and IFA testing of the brain for rabies antigen were negative. Histopathologic findings were consistent with FIP.

191 A 9-year-old castrated male Siamese mix was referred for examination of stomatitis (191a). The cat was known to be infected with FIV for at least 6 years. A biopsy of the gingival tissue was consistent with lymphoplasmacytic stomatitis.

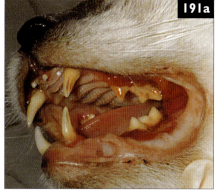

i. What is the pathogenesis of stomatitis in FIV infection?
ii. What treatment is most likely to resolve the condition permanently?
A. Treatment with antibiotics such as amoxicillin/clavulanate or clindamycin.
B. Treatment with azithromycin for bartonellosis.
C. Dental scaling and polishing with extraction of decayed teeth.
D. Full-mouth dental extraction.
E. Immunosuppressive dosages of prednisolone and/or cyclosporin.

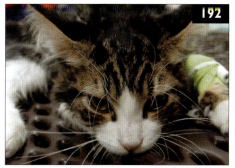

192 A 5-year-old domestic shorthair cat was seen because of sudden-onset lethargy of 1 day's duration (192). On physical examination, pale and icteric oral mucous membranes, weak peripheral pulses, and a body temperature of 36.5°C were noted. Additionally, the cat appeared to have diffuse abdominal pain. The respiratory rate (66 bpm) and heart rate (240 bpm) were increased, and the systolic blood pressure (85 mmHg) was decreased. The cat was suspected to be in endotoxemic shock.
i. What is endotoxin?
ii. Is it possible to have a negative blood culture in an endotoxemic patient?
iii. What are risk factors for endotoxemia in the cat?

191 i. Up to 50% of FIV-infected cats may suffer from chronic ulceroproliferative stomatitis. It characteristically originates in the fauces and gradually spreads rostrally, especially along the maxillary teeth. Pain and tooth loss are common, and severe stomatitis can lead to anorexia and emaciation. The cause is uncertain, although the histologic findings suggest an immune response to chronic antigenic stimulation, or immune dysregulation. In addition, circulating lymphocytes of cats with stomatitis have higher than normal expression

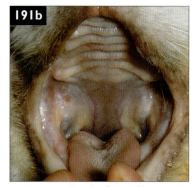

of inflammatory cytokines, further implicating immune activation in the pathogenesis. Concurrent FCV infection is often identified and may be a cofactor inducing stomatitis along with FIV. Other infectious agents may also play a role.

ii. D. Full-mouth dental extraction. In some cats with inflammation limited to the fauces, the canine and incisor teeth may be left *in situ*. Particular attention must be paid to complete removal of all tooth roots. Therefore, dental radiographs should be performed after the end of the procedure. Other treatments may partially palliate the gingival inflammation (although immunosupressants should be avoided in FIV-infected cats), but extraction is usually required to resolve the disease permanently. The prognosis for a full recovery is better for FIV-infected cats than for FIV-negative cats. Full-mouth dental extraction followed by a 2-week course of amoxicillin/clavulanate resulted in complete resolution of the stomatitis in this cat (**191b**).

192 i. Endotoxin is lipopolysaccharide (LPS) released from the outer membrane of lysed Gram-negative bacteria. In a healthy individual, endotoxin associated with ingesta or intestinal flora is cleared by the gut-associated immune system and the portal circulation. The organisms usually implicated are *Pseudomonas* spp., *Escherichia* spp., *Klebsiella* spp., *Enterbacter* spp., and *Proteus* spp.

ii. In some cases of endotoxemia, viable bacteria are present in the blood leading to positive blood cultures, but endotoxemic cats can have negative blood cultures. Bacteria may remain compartmentalized in the tissues or intestine or may be nonviable, resulting in negative blood cultures.

iii. Risk factors for sepsis and endotoxemia in cats include bite wounds, septic peritonitis, pyothorax, and bacteremia secondary to pyelonephritis, gastrointestinal disease, pneumonia, endocarditis, osteomyelitis, and pyometra. Icterus associated with sepsis and endotoxemia is often a result of cholestasis in the absence of structural hepatic disease or hepatic infection.

193 A 12-year-old castrated male domestic shorthair cat was seen because of weight loss, dropping food while eating, poor coat, lower energy than previously, and halitosis (193). On physical examination, severe periodontal disease was noted with a region of marked inflammation on one side of the mandible. The man-

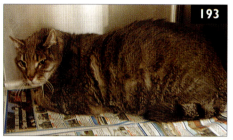

dibular lymph node on the same side was enlarged, and a small draining fistula was seen adjacent to one tooth in the area.
i. How does osteomyelitis develop?
ii. Which organisms may play a role?
iii. How do acute and chronic osteomyelitis differ in presentation?
iv. What treatment is recommended for this cat?

194 A 1-year-old intact female Himalayan cat was seen because of depression and rapid breathing. The cat lived exclusively indoors, was managed holistically without vaccinations, and was fed a diet supplemented with raw meat. On physical examination, the cat was tachypneic (55 bpm), had high body temperature (40.0°C), and dull mentation (194a). There was increased inspiratory effort and bronchovesicular sounds in all lung fields. Ophthalmic examination revealed bilateral ocular lesions (194b).
i. What are the rule-outs for high body temperature?
ii. What is the abnormality seen on fundic examination?

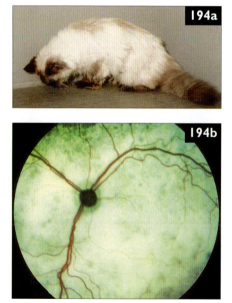

193 i. Normal bone is resistant to infection. However, ischemia, bacterial contamination, the presence of foreign material, bone necrosis and sequestration, and changes in the local or systemic immune response may all play a role in the development of osteomyelitis.

ii. Several reports indicate that *Staphylococcus* spp. account for up to 60% of all bacterial cases. *Streptococcus* and *Enterococcus* spp. are other Gram-positive organisms that may be implicated. Gram-negative organisms are also implicated and include *Pasteurella*, *E. coli*, and *Pseudomonas* spp. Anerobes that have been cultured include *Actinomyces*, *Nocardia*, and *Bacteroides* and isolation of these fastidious agents has increased with improved sample handling. Fungal organisms may also cause osteomyelitis.

iii. Acute osteomyelitis often presents with fever, localized pain, erythema, swelling, lethargy, and leukocytosis. As the condition becomes chronic, a draining tract, lameness, or ill thrift may be the only findings.

iv. The cat should be anesthetized for teeth cleaning including subgingival curettage, individual tooth examination including periodontal probing to evaluate and chart pocket depths, polishing, radiography of affected teeth, and biopsy of the affected bone for histology and culture to determine whether the affected area is neoplastic or infected. Establishment of drainage and debridement to remove ischemic, necrotic tissue is critical for optimal healing along with treatment with antimicrobials appropriate for the agent. Antimicrobials chosen must be safe for long-term use, must reach therapeutic levels in bone, and must be based on culture and sensitivity results. Most often, these results will show organism susceptibility to first-generation cephalosporins, amoxicillin/clavulanate; for Gram-negative aerobes, quinolones, second/third-generation cephalosporins, imipenem, or ticaracillin/clavulanate may be required. With anerobic organisms, amoxicillin/clavulanate, metronidazole, or clindamycin may be effective. Antibiotics should be continued for at least 3 weeks past clinical resolution of osteomyelitis. In the case of routine treatment of periodontal disease, cats should receive antibiotics IV immediately prior to dental prophylaxis because 36% of cats with periodontal disease undergoing prophylaxis have positive blood cultures at the time of dental prophylaxis. In this case, there was less redness in the mouth 2 weeks after dental prophylaxis. Antibiotics were continued for another month, at which time the cat had improved greatly. Six months later, there was no apparent recurrence of the clinical signs of infection.

194 i. The two rule-outs for high body temperature are fever or hyperthermia. Fever is more likely in this case as causes of hyperthermia (stress, overheating, hyperthyroidism) were unlikely. The most common causes of fever are infectious inflammation, noninfectious inflammation (e.g. autoimmune diseases), and neoplasia.

ii. There is evidence of chorioretinitis in this cat.

195 Case 195 is the same cat as case 194.

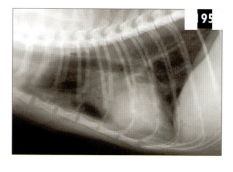

Blood profile/ biochemistry panel	Results
Hematocrit	0.27 l/l
Neutrophilia	$16.5 \times 10^9/l$
Left shift band neutrophils	$0.85 \times 10^9/l$
Lymphocytosis	$8.1 \times 10^9/l$
Monocytosis	$1.20 \times 10^9/l$
ALT – increased	255 IU/l
ALP – increased	156 IU/l

Thoracic radiographs (195) were taken.
i. What is the radiographic interpretation?
ii. What is the next diagnostic step?

196 Case 196 is the same cat as cases 194 and 195. A BAL was performed through a sterile endotracheal tube. A cytologic preparation was evaluated (196) (Wrights–Giemsa stain).
i. What is the diagnosis?
ii. What treatment should be provided?
iii. How did the cat probably acquire the infection?

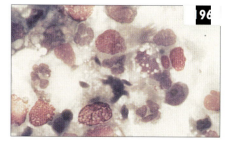

197 A 10-year-old neutered female domestic shorthair cat was seen because of ocular disease and anorexia. Physical examination revealed weight loss, lethargy, anorexia, generalized lymphadenopathy, symmetric alopecia on the ear pinnae with nodular dermatitis, and bilateral ocular changes (197). Previous treatment consisted of amoxicillin/ clavulanate for 7 days but had not led to any improvement.
i. How can the ocular changes be characterized, and what are the differential diagnoses for this clinical picture?
ii. What should the diagnostic plan be?

195 i. There is a patchy interstitial alveolar pattern of the lungs.
ii. Collection of BAL fluid for cytology and culture is indicated.

196 i. There is a mixed inflammatory reaction predominated by neutrophils and macrophages. Several small basophilic banana-shaped organisms consistent with *Toxoplasma gondii* tachyzoites are present. The cat has toxoplasmosis of the lungs with widespread dissemination to the CNS and other organs likely.
ii. The drug of choice is clindamycin given at a high dose (10.0–12.5 mg/kg PO q 12 h) for 4 weeks. Clinical improvement is expected to begin within the first days of treatment. Severely affected cats may experience an early period of deterioration due to increased inflammatory responses shortly after initiation of therapy. These cats may benefit from anti-inflammatory dosages of prednisolone for a few days. Prolonged use of immunosuppressive drugs should be avoided. Therapy was uncomplicated in this cat and there was complete recovery from clinical signs. It should be remembered that once an individual has recovered from toxoplasmosis, inactive tissue cysts remain present for life and may be reactivated during immunosuppression.
iii. Cats typically acquire toxoplasmosis from hunting diseased animals or consuming contaminated raw meat. In this indoor cat, the source was probably the raw meat diet. The risk of toxoplasmosis can be reduced by feeding commercial cooked diets, cooking meat, or freezing meat to lower than –12°C for at least 24 hours.

197 i. The cat shows a bilateral uveitis with aqueous flare, iritis, hyphema, and hypopion. The fundic examination revealed small hemorrhages and posterior synechia. The most common causes of bilateral uveitis are systemic diseases (e.g. infectious, neoplastic). In intraocular bleeding of undetermined cause, a neoplasm always has to be considered. Lymphoma is the most common tumor of the eyes of cats and usually demonstrates aqueous flare, iris swelling, changes in iris color, and iris vascularization. Infectious diseases can be caused by viral, bacterial, fungal, and parasitic infections. The most common infectious agents include FCoV, FeLV, FIV, *Toxoplasma gondii*, *Bartonella* spp., and fungi (e.g. cryptococcosis, histoplasmosis). In endemic areas unusual systemic diseases (e.g. leishmaniasis, ehrlichiosis) also have to be considered.
ii. Investigation into the cause of the uveitis includes complete blood count, biochemistry panel, urinalysis, and tests for infectious diseases (e.g. FeLV, FIV, fungi, *T. gondii*). Tests for leishmaniasis and ehrlichiosis are necessary in endemic areas. Examination of aqueous humor and detection of local antibodies (e.g. against *T. gondii*, *Bartonella* spp., fungi) is also an option, and antibodies detected in aqueous humor are better suited for establishing a diagnosis than antibodies in the serum.

198 Case **198** is the same cat as case **197**. The cat had severe uveitis (**198**).

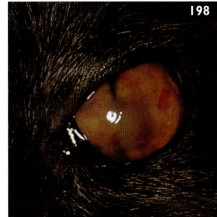

Blood profile/ biochemistry panel	Results
Hematocrit – mild nonregenerative anemia	0.29 l/l
Leukopenia	4.3 × 10⁹/l
Hyperproteinemia	91 g/l
Hypoalbuminemia	18 g/l
Hyperglobulinemia	73 g/l
Albumin : globulin	0.25

Serum electrophoresis showed a polyclonal gammopathy. Urinalysis was unremarkable. FeLV antigen, FIV antibody, and *T. gondii* IgM and IgG antibody tests were negative. The *Leishmania* spp. antibody titer was 1:128 (high titer).
i. How can these results be interpreted?
ii. What tests should be done next?

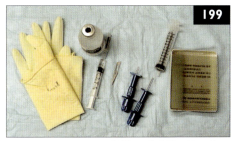

199 Case **199** is the same cat as cases **197** and **198**. Cytology of aqueous humor showed primarily macrophages with rare round basophilic nuclei suggestive of amastigotes. A bone marrow aspirate was collected (**199**). Bone marrow cytology and bone marrow PCR confirmed the presence of *Leishmania* spp.
i. What is the diagnostic value of antibody testing and PCR for the diagnosis of leishmaniasis?
ii. What is the *Leishmania* spp. antibody prevalence in cats in endemic areas?

198 i. Mild nonregenerative anemia in cats is most commonly caused by chronic inflammation (e.g. systemic infections, neoplasms). Tests for detection of antibodies against *Leishmania* spp. in cats are not very reliable. The presence of antibodies is not diagnostic for the disease since positive results can occur in healthy cats as well as diseased cats. In addition, in countries in which leishmaniasis has been reported in cats (Asia, South America, USA, the Mediterranean area including Spain, Portugal, Italy, and France) less than 50% of the diseased cats have antibodies against *Leishmania* spp.
ii. Further diagnostics should include bone marrow aspiration for cytology and PCR for *Leishmania* spp. on blood and bone marrow samples. In addition, cytology can be performed on an imprint or aspirate of the pinna lesions. In doubtful cases, immunohistochemical techniques can be used to stain the organism. PCR testing of aqueous humor may be useful.

199 i. Antibody testing for leishmaniasis is generally less reliable in cats than in dogs because many cats that are infected do not have detectable antibodies. The antibody titers appear to be lower in affected cats than in dogs, although the number of clinical cases is small. PCR of bone marrow samples is the most reliable test to diagnose the disease. PCR tests on feline blood samples are in progress but preliminary results confirm the presence of *Leishmania* DNA in such speciments.
ii. Antibody prevalence against *Leishmania* spp. in cats from endemic areas varies widely. In one study, only 1 of 110 (0.9%) cat serum samples collected in Italy examined by immunofluorescent antibody (IFA) and in another study only 14 of 175 (8%) samples tested by enzyme-linked immunofluorescent assay (ELISA) and Western blot were positive for anti-*Leishmania* spp. antibodies. However, other studies performed in Italy and Spain using IFA showed an antibody prevalence of between 42 and 59%. In some endemic areas serological surveys have also been carried out in cats, using IHAT in Egypt, Western blot in France, and IFAT in Italy. Sixty Egyptian cats had low serological antibody titers, from 1/32 to 1/128; in the endemic focus of canine leishmaniasis of Alpes Maritimes, 12 out of 97 (12.5%) cats showed antibodies versus antigens of *L. infantum*. Regardless of the actual prevalence of infection, leishmaniasis should be included in the differential diagnosis of systemic and/or dermatologic diseases in endemic areas. The cat should be considered an animal with an active role in the transmission and diffusion of leishmaniasis, unlike goats, calves, and horses that could serve as accidental reservoirs of the disease. In fact it has been demonstrated that some feline parasites (*Phlebotomus perniciosus*) act as vectors of *L. infantum*, suggesting that cats may represent an additional domestic reservoir for this protoza.

Table of reference ranges

(SI units and conventional units) in adult cats
(in cats, some values (*) can be increased in stress)

Physical examination	Reference interval (SI units)	Reference interval (conventional units)	Conversion factor (SI to conventional units)
Body weight	*variable* (kg)	*variable* (lb)	2.2
Body temperature	38.0–39.0* (°C)	100–102* (°F)	1.8 (+ 32)
Heart rate	120–180* (bpm)	120–180* (bpm)	1
Respiratory rate	20–40* (bpm)	20–40* (bpm)	1
Systolic blood pressure	100–160* (mmHg)	100–160* (mmHg)	1

Complete blood count	Reference interval (SI units)	Reference interval (conventional units)	Conversion factor (SI to conventional units)
Red blood cells	5–10 (× 10^{12}/l)	5–10 (× 10^6/µl)	1
Hemoglobin	5.5–10.5 (mmol/l)	8.8–16.9 (g/dl)	0.6206
Hematocrit	0.30–0.45 (l/l)	30–45%	0.01
MCV	40–55 (fl)	40–55 (fl)	1
MCH	0.8–1.0 (fmol/l)	0.8–1.0 (pg)	1
MCHC	19–22 (mmol/l)	19–22 (mmol/l)	1
Reticulocytes	0–60 (× 10^9/l)	0–60 (× 10^3/µl)	1
Platelets	200–600 (× 10^9/l)	200–600 (× 10^3/µl)	1
MPV	11–18 (fl)	11–18 (fl)	1
White blood cells	5–18* (× 10^9/l)	5–18* (× 10^3/µl)	1
Mature neutrophils	3–11* (× 10^9/l)	3–11* (× 10^3/µl)	1
Band neutrophils	0–0.4 (× 10^9/l)	0–0.4 (× 10^3/µl)	1
Eosinophils	0–1.0 (× 10^9/l)	0–1.0 (× 10^3/µl)	1
Basophils	0–0.4 (× 10^9/l)	0–0.4 (× 10^3/µl)	1
Lymphocytes	1.5–7.0 (× 10^9/l)	1.5–7.0 (× 10^3/µl)	1
Monocytes	0–1.0 (× 10^9/l)	0–1.0 (× 10^3/µl)	1

Table of reference ranges

Coagulation panel	Reference interval (SI units)	Reference interval (conventional units)	Conversion factor (SI to conventional units)
PT	0–8 (sec)	0–8 (sec)	1
PTT	0–13 (sec)	0–13 (sec)	1
TT	0–12 (sec)	0–12 (sec)	1
Antithrombin III	95–130 (%)	95–130 (%)	1
FDP	0–20 (μg/ml)	0–20 (μg/ml)	1

Biochemistry panel	Reference interval (SI units)	Reference interval (conventional units)	Conversion factor (SI to conventional units)
ALT	0–100 (IU/l)	0–100 (IU/l)	1
ALP	0–50 (IU/l)	0 – 50 (IU/l)	1
GDH	0–10 (IU/l)	0–10 (IU/l)	1
γ-GT	0–5 (IU/l)	0–5 (IU/l)	1
AST	0–50 (IU/l)	0–50 (IU/l)	1
CK	0–400 (IU/l)	0–400 (IU/l)	1
LDH	0–300 (IU/l)	0–300 (IU/l)	1
α-Amylase	0–2000 (IU/l)	0–2000 (IU/l)	1
Lipase	0–300 (IU/l)	0–300 (IU/l)	1
Cholinesterase	2300–4500 (IU/l)	2300–4500 (IU/l)	1
Total protein	55–80 (g/l)	5.5–8.0 (g/dl)	0.1
Albumin	25–40 (g/l)	2.5–4.0 (g/dl)	0.1
Globulins	25–50 (g/l)	2.5–5.0 (g/dl)	0.1
Bilirubin	0–5 (μmol/l)	0–0.3 (mg/dl)	0.059
Bile acids	0–20 (μmol/l)	0–8 (μg/ml)	0.41
NH_3	0–60 (μmol/l)	0–60 (μEq/l)	1
Creatinine	0 – 170 (μmol/l)	0 – 1.9 (mg/dl)	0.0113
Urea	5–10 (mmol/l)	14–28 (mg/dl BUN)	2.8
Glucose	4–7* (mmol/l)	72–126* (mg/dl)	18
Sodium	145–155 (mmol/l)	145–155 (mEq/l)	1
Potassium	3.5–5.5 (mmol/l)	3.5–5.5 (mEq/l)	1
Chloride	110–130 (mmol/l)	110–130 (mEq/l)	1
Calcium	2.1–2.6 (mmol/l)	8.4–10.4 (mg/dl)	4
Phosphate	1.0–2.3 (mmol/l)	3.1–7.1 (mg/dl)	3.1
Magnesium	0.7–2.6 (mmol/l)	0.7–2.6 (mmol/l)	1
TCO_2	17–24 (mmol/l)	17–24 (mEq/l)	1
Anion gap	8–19 (mval/l)	8–19 (mval/l)	1

Table of reference ranges

Urinalysis	Reference interval (SI units)	Reference interval (conventional units)	Conversion factor (SI to conventional units)
Color, appearance	yellow, clear	yellow, clear	–
Specific gravity	1.001–1.080	1.001–1.080	1
pH	5–7	5–7	1
Protein	–	–	–
Glucose	–	–	–
Ketone	–	–	–
Bilirubin	–	–	–
Blood	–	–	–
Protein to creatinine ratio	0–0.5	0–0.5	1
Red blood cells	0–5 (/hpf)	0–5 (/hpf)	1
White blood cells	0–3 (/hpf)	0–3 (/hpf)	1
Casts	0 (/hpf)	0 (/hpf)	1

Index

Note: locator numbers refer to case numbers

Index

Index